The Integrated Medical Curriculum

The Integrated Medical Curriculum

RAJA C BANDARANAYAKE

MBBS, PhD, MSEd, FRACS
Consultant in Medical Education
Former Associate Professor & Director (Academic), School of Medical Education
University of New South Wales, Sydney
Former Professor of Anatomy, Arabian Gulf University, Bahrain

Forewords by

STEPHEN ABRAHAMSON

PhD, ScD
Professor Emeritus of Medical Education
Founding Chair, Department of Medical Education
Former Associate Dean for Medical Education
University of Southern California School of Medicine
Los Angeles

and

RONALD HARDEN

OBE, MD, FRCP (GLAS.), FRCS (ED.), FRCPC
General Secretary, Association for Medical Education in Europe
Professor, Centre for Medical Education
University of Dundee

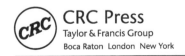

CRC Press
Taylor & Francis Group
Boca Raton London New York

CRC Press is an imprint of the
Taylor & Francis Group, an **informa** business

Radcliffe Publishing Ltd
33–41 Dallington Street
London
EC1V 0BB
United Kingdom

www.radcliffepublishing.com
Electronic catalogue and worldwide online ordering facility.

British Library Cataloguing in Publication Data

A catalogue record for this book is available from the British Library.

ISBN-13: 978 184619 510 5

The paper used for the text pages of this book is FSC® certified. FSC (The Forest Stewardship Council®) is an international network to promote responsible management of the world's forests.

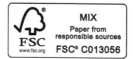

Typeset by Pindar NZ, Auckland, New Zealand

Contents

Foreword by Stephen Abrahamson

The history of American medical education may provide some insights into the almost incredible slowness of change. This book has referred to some of that history and a few more comments might help the reader understand better the value and importance of this work on integrated curriculum for medical and other health professional schools.

It is interesting, for instance, to discover that the American Medical Association (AMA) was founded in 1847 because physicians in the United States were concerned about the education and training of young people for the practice of medicine. Only later did the AMA evolve into its present role as a lobbying group working primarily for the economic interests and concerns of physicians. But in the mid nineteenth century, the major concern was the standardisation and improvement of medical education. And it is interesting to note that it was in 1893 that the importance of basic sciences in the practice of medicine was recognised by the faculty of the Johns Hopkins School of Medicine – that happening contributed greatly to the improvement of medical education in the United States.

However, it was also the beginning of the growth of a problem, well discussed by the author, which has grown troublesome since its inception: the separation of basic sciences from the clinical disciplines. Basic sciences were seen as necessary bodies of information *before* studying the clinical applications of those bodies of knowledge. And, as the basic science information bases grew with the 'explosion of knowledge' during the several decades in the middle of the twentieth century, more and more emphasis was placed on medical students having to learn those 'bodies of knowledge'. Furthermore, as this book tells us, experts in those basic sciences were sought to teach that knowledge, unfortunately by asking students to memorise the information.

At the next level of medical education, the clinical disciplines, similar problems grew out of the vast new knowledge areas being 'discovered' through research in speciality areas. Thus, the two major areas of speciality (basic sciences and clinical disciplines) were divided internally into smaller and smaller specialities with stronger and stronger special interest groups.

Meanwhile, the Flexner Report in 1910 laid out a basic plan for a medical school curriculum that, in the United States, was not challenged until the curriculum change at Western Reserve University (now Case Western Reserve University) School of Medicine. At the heart of that change, cordially rejected by the vast majority of American medical schools, was the first recognition that the basic sciences should be learnt not as separate bodies of information but as intrinsically related to each other, and that they should be learnt in the context of clinical problems.

The negative reaction was purely a question of guarding one's academic 'turf', and has been seen as the primary reaction to many other attempts at making changes to improve medical education, perhaps most notably the introduction of a problem-based curriculum at McMaster University's School of Medicine in Canada. Mentioned by the author, this change was thoroughly rejected by most American medical schools until Harvard University developed its own problem-based curriculum, and this was followed by other medical schools' investigations of the area. However, these schools did not have a carefully designed plan to follow for the development and implementation of such a new curriculum. This book presents a carefully thought-out rationale for an 'integrated curriculum' and an equally well thought-out plan for the implementation of such a curriculum.

Readers are urged to consider carefully the setting (their own respective medical school) as they come to understand the rationale and implementation. Their use of the rationale and implementation plan must be carefully applied for success. But clearly, all of the steps are presented.

One final note is the recognition of the author, Dr Raja Bandaranayake, as a remarkably well-qualified person to present this work. His broad experience, along with his intensive study of medical education, has made him well qualified to design the curriculum and describe its application steps.

Stephen Abrahamson PhD, ScD
Professor Emeritus of Medical Education
Founding Chair, Department of Medical Education
Former Associate Dean for Medical Education
University of Southern California School of Medicine
Los Angeles
January 2011

Foreword by Ronald Harden

The SPICES model for analysing and planning a medical curriculum, as I described it in 1984, embodies key educational strategies. *Student-centredness* was an obvious feature. Who could object to the idea that the student was at the centre of the learning process and that what mattered was what the students learnt and not what the teacher taught? For the most part, however, only lip service has been paid to the concept although with the development of the internet and new learning technologies increasing attention is being paid to independent learning. The future perhaps holds more promise for a student-centred curriculum featuring adaptive learning tailored to meet the needs of individual students. *Problem-based* learning attracted much attention and over the years has been adopted in an increasing number of schools. At the same time the approach has attracted criticism and some schools who were initially strong proponents now appear to be less enthusiastic. *Community-based* education has been slow to be recognised but undoubtedly, in line with patients' expectations and political pressures, it will become an increasingly important focus for attention albeit if only a peripheral interest in many medical schools. *Electives* or student-selected courses bring with them significant benefits but inevitably play only a relatively minor role in the typical medical curriculum. A *systematic* approach with an emphasis on outcome-based education is a recent curriculum initiative of significance although its impact on practice has still to be demonstrated. Of the six education strategies described in the SPICES model, *integration* has taken centre stage. An integrated approach is now the basis for the curriculum in schools around the world although there are geographical differences with a discipline-based approach still featuring as the norm in some countries.

Over the last half century around the world there has been an increasing emphasis on an integrated approach in medical education. In the United Kingdom, the General Medical Council stated in 1957 that '[i]t is desirable that interdepartmental teaching should be encouraged throughout the whole period of professional study'. By 1967 the Council were more positive:

The Council would also like to encourage [interdisciplinary teaching] through-out the undergraduate curriculum. Stimulating in itself, it (interdisciplinary teaching) serves to demonstrate that, although it is convenient and in many respects helpful that separate departments should be responsible for the vari-ous subjects of the curriculum, the subjects nevertheless cannot without loss be compartmentalised in teaching.

There was also, however, a reservation: 'This has the one disadvantage that it is expensive of teaching time. It cannot therefore be extravagantly employed'. By 1993 the position taken by the General Medical Council on integration was more positive and required that '[t]he core curriculum should be *system-based*, its component parts being the combined responsibility of basic scientists and clinicians *integrating* their contributions to a common purpose, thus eliminat-ing the rigid pre-clinical/clinical divide and the exclusive departmentally based course'.

To begin with there was wide opposition to the adoption of an integrated cur-riculum. Writing in the *Lancet* (1964, i, 283), Sir Charles Illingworth, Professor of Surgery at the University of Glasgow, highlighted the resistance to change and the conservatism of the medical establishment:

Medical schools are not designed for change. They are feudal kingdoms where every baron is all-powerful in his own castle. Every professor agrees in principle with the need for pruning the curriculum, but the prestige and genuine belief in the importance of his own subject impel him to demand extra lecture time for his own department.

As a student at the University of Glasgow in the 1950s, my medical studies con-sisted of a series of departmentally based courses, each with its own syllabus and examination. Joining the Glasgow Medical School in the 1960s as a lecturer in medicine, I was given responsibility for introducing a new integrated course with a custom-built integrated teaching suite. This followed the model of an organ-system integrated curriculum introduced at Western Reserve University (now Case Western Reserve University) in the 1950s where the curriculum was more closely aligned with the knowledge base used by physicians in practice. Despite some initial opposition, the advantages of the integrated approach became obvi-ous to teachers and students. The expansion of knowledge and the pressure for new subjects to be included in the curriculum had been a recognised problem that the integrated approach now addressed. Staff from different departments were encouraged to work together to determine what content was relevant and important and the appropriate level of depth at which it should be studied. The integrated approach in the new Glasgow curriculum encouraged conceptual inte-gration and the development of higher-level objectives. An undoubted additional benefit was that staff from different disciplines were brought together, often for the first time, to share their common interests and collaborative research activities were stimulated.

In 1972 I moved from Glasgow to the University of Dundee where I was charged, working with the Curriculum Committee, to revitalise what was very much a departmentally based curriculum. Strong proponents for change were the students. Some years earlier, in 1965, in 'A Report on Medical Education, Suggestions for the Future' the British Medical Students Association had argued:

> In spite of the tremendous advances in medical knowledge and practice, the form of medical education has remained virtually static over the last hundred years with new subjects grudgingly being given teaching space within the curriculum, many years after they should have been. This has resulted in gross overcrowding of the curriculum which has been divided into isolated compartments by the departments responsible for teaching. An end must be put to this. . . . the medical school departments must co-operate with each other to produce a fully integrated, yet flexible, curriculum.

The discussion about the introduction of the integrated curriculum in Dundee included the terminology to be used. Given some resistance to the concept of 'integration' the term 'coordinated systematic course' was adopted. The disadvantages of a traditional discipline-based approach to medical education with the resulting fragmentation of learning had become apparent and departments agreed to pool their resources to create an integrated teaching programme. The integrated Dundee curriculum continued to evolve in response to the changing needs and with each subsequent curriculum review the concept of integration was endorsed and the curriculum seen as 'a curriculum where the whole was greater than the sum of the parts'. Vertical integration was strengthened with a spiral curriculum where students progressed to new levels of the spiral with information introduced that linked directly back to information from previous phases of the curriculum. By this time in the 1970s integration was on the medical education agenda and almost two-thirds of medical schools in the United Kingdom had an integrated curriculum or planned to introduce one. One school, however, had reported discontinuing an integrated curriculum and another had rejected the approach for logistical reasons. Developments with integrated curricula were taking place around the world. Over the remainder of the twentieth century, integration became a recognised and established approach to the curriculum globally with development of the concept expanding to embrace ideas such as interprofessional education.

It can be argued, with some conviction, that of the different educational strategies integration has had the greatest impact on medical education. Integration is a powerful concept and might even be described as a new vision that emerged for teaching and learning in medicine. A key feature was the importance attached to authentic learning with the students' learning related to the real-life context. Today the reigning curriculum model in medicine is the integrated curriculum, most commonly organised around organ systems.

What is meant by an integrated curriculum and how integration is delivered in practice, however, is a somewhat contested area. I have previously described 11 steps on what I have called 'an integration ladder'. Each step has attracted its own and varied terminology. A textbook on the subject by a leading authority in medical education who can write not only from a theoretical perspective but also from his own experience in curriculum planning in countries around the world is to be welcomed. Raja Bandaranayake demonstrates a thorough grasp of the subject and, from his own experience in the area and from delivering staff development programmes on the topic, is well equipped to provide all stakeholders with a rich understanding of integration. *The Integrated Medical Curriculum* helps readers to understand the concept of an integrated curriculum, to appreciate the underpinning of educational theory and potential advantages and related problems and to familiarise themselves with issues arising from the implementation of an integrated approach in practice. The author clarifies some of the mysteries surrounding integration and addresses a number of important issues. He emphasises that there is no universal model of integration. Indeed, the text is unusual to the extent that it offers not one but a range of integration frameworks and encourages the reader to make informed decisions in their own setting once they are aware of and understand the options. It recognises that there can be problems and real tensions associated with implementing an integrated approach but that these can be tackled positively.

Albert Einstein wrote 'any intelligent fool can make things bigger, more complex, and more violent . . .. it takes a touch of genius – and a lot of courage – to move in the opposite direction'. Raja Bandaranayake has taken a difficult and multifaceted subject and, without losing any of the more subtle nuances and difficulties, has made it appear simple. Important issues he has addressed include the focus for the integration – should the curriculum be integrated around a body system, a theme or stage in the life cycle or a set of patient problems? He emphasises the importance of avoiding a mismatch between teaching and assessment. I remember sitting in the back of a lecture theatre in one school I visited listening to an integrated lecture and finding students writing in several notebooks. I asked the students whether this was to provide notes for their colleagues who were unable to be present at the lecture but I was corrected. Apparently although the course was integrated the examination was not and students were writing in one book matters relating to medicine, in another book surgery-related facts and in a third book information relating to pharmacology. Another issue addressed is the learning resources that are available to support an integrated course. Many text books are discipline- or subject-based but, particularly with the increasing availability of resources online, this is changing. Who should be responsible for the integration in an integrated curriculum – the student or the teacher? While this task normally falls to the teacher, the student can also be actively engaged. This is certainly so where a task-based approach is adopted. Here students have as a basis for their learning a set of tasks such as the management of abdominal pain. As students pass through the clinical attachments it is their responsibility to look at how each contributes to their learning. In the medical attachment their learning may relate to the presentation and investigation of a patient with abdominal pain, in the surgical attachment to the management of acute abdominal pain, in the obstetrics and gynaecology attachment the management of abdominal pain in women, in the paediatric attachment to abdominal pain in children and in the general practice attachment to issues relating to uncertainty in medicine where no diagnosis is made and to the indications for referring a patient for more detailed investigation.

Bandaranayake argues that the most common deterrent to successful integration is a lack of a correct and shared understanding by faculty of the concept of integration. This book will help faculty to move from their comfort zone of departments and subjects and encourage them to adopt an integrated approach without fear of territorial loss or harm to their students' learning. It provides practical advice and guidelines that, if followed, should lead to the successful adoption of an integrated approach to the curriculum with all the associated benefits. Integration once regarded as an innovation in medical education is now an established feature of the medical curriculum. This book helps us to understand how this happened and what it means for teachers, course leaders, deans, researchers, administrators and, importantly, for students.

Ronald Harden OBE, MD, FRCP (GLAS.), FRCS (ED.), FRCPC
General Secretary, Association for Medical Education in Europe
Professor, Centre for Medical Education
University of Dundee
January 2011

Preface

The pioneering curriculum change that occurred in Western Reserve University School of Medicine in 1952, from a discipline-based curriculum to an organ-systems-based, integrated one, should have stimulated other medical schools to make a similar change. However, this did not occur. Some schools were willing to include integrated components in their curricula, but neither the basic nature of the curriculum nor the stranglehold that the departments held in the organisational structure of the school changed significantly over the next half century.

In 1968 McMaster University's School of Medicine pioneered a method of curriculum integration through problem-based learning, with interdepartmental committees controlling the teaching programme. Though a few schools in different parts of the world were at first willing to follow this lead, once again a trend was not created until the final decade of the last century and the first decade of the present century, when there was a significant and rapid increase in the number of schools that adopted this strategy in some part of the curriculum. Many schools, however, continue to be sceptical about such a major reorientation of not only the curriculum but also the entire fabric of the medical school. Many are still to be convinced that the basic structure of the school should be rearranged to accommodate this change.

The relatively recent spurt of activity in relation to the medical curriculum may, perhaps, be attributed to the exhortations of international and national bodies for medical schools to consider curriculum integration seriously.

The Australian Medical Council (AMC) in 1998, referring to the body responsible for curriculum design, implementation and student assessment, urged that 'membership of this committee should include the basic and clinical sciences.[1] It recommended basic science teaching be based around clinical problems, and clinicians to be more involved in teaching basic sciences.

In 2003, the World Federation for Medical Education promulgated its global standards for basic medical education, one of which was that 'basic sciences and clinical sciences should be integrated in the curriculum [and] integration of disciplines would include both horizontal (concurrent) and vertical (sequential) integration of curricular components'. It also recommended that 'examinations should be adjusted by integrating assessment of various curricular elements to encourage integrated learning'.[2]

In the most recent issue of its guidelines, published in June 2010, the Liaison Committee on Medical Education for medical schools in the United States and Canada recommended that 'content is coordinated and integrated within and across academic periods of study [and that] the structure and content of courses and clinical attachments should integrate learning about basic medical sciences and clinical sciences'. In addition they urged medical schools to 'ensure that students work with and learn from other health and social care professionals and students [so that they] understand the importance of teamwork in providing care'.[3]

In its 2009 version of the document *Tomorrow's Doctors*, the General Medical Council in the United Kingdom stipulates, as one of its criteria for developing undergraduate curricula, the following: 'The curriculum will be structured to provide a balance of learning opportunities and to integrate the learning of basic and clinical sciences, enabling students to link theory and practice'.[4]

The Gulf Cooperation Council Medical Colleges Deans' Committee, in laying down its recommendations and guidelines on minimum standards for establishing and accrediting medical schools in 2001, stated that '[a]n appropriate level of horizontal (concurrent) and vertical (sequential) integration must be in place in order to achieve the educational objectives'. To this end,

> basic science courses must illustrate the importance of principles being taught to the understanding of health and disease, both at the individual and community level [and] clinical science must be taught in such a way that the underlying scientific principles and humanitarian values are reinforced.[5]

It is clear that national bodies responsible for accrediting medical curricula in their respective countries, as well as a world body on whose standards many other countries base their accrediting procedures, place great emphasis on curriculum integration. A cursory glance at the proceedings of a recent Asia-Pacific medical education conference revealed that representatives of at least 10 countries in the region presented the efforts they were taking to introduce integrated curricula of one form or another in their schools.[6]

In spite of these exhortations and efforts, it is still true that the majority of medical curricula continue to be discipline-based. This does not mean that these curricula are not integrated. The danger, however, is that as teachers become increasingly entrenched in their own disciplines they tend not to see beyond the narrow confines of those disciplines, and the victim is the student, who learns to satisfy immediate needs rather than the ultimate goal of healthcare, which transcends disciplinary boundaries.

This book caters to those who are desirous of improving their curricula, their separate courses or even their individual teaching endeavours to produce a physician who is accustomed to displaying integrating behaviour when confronted with community or clinical problems in professional life. It also caters to the needs of those who are engaged in the task of advising others to do so. Lastly, it meets the needs of the serious student of curriculum theory and practice, as an increasing number of graduate and postgraduate courses in education for the health professions take their rightful place in the offerings of many tertiary educational institutions.

In Chapter 1, a philosophical consideration of the nature of integration in general, and of integration of learning more specifically, is followed by a discussion of how learning theory influences the curriculum. The thoughts expressed by some leading educational psychologists help to examine the concept of integration in relation to the curriculum.

In tracing the history of the integrated medical curriculum in Chapter 2, the factors that led to its introduction, particularly the unbridled growth of the specialities, are discussed. The introduction of problem-based learning in medical education was triggered by developments in secondary education, while the marriage of the art and science of medicine arose from a realisation that medical education was moving rapidly away from the former.

In Chapter 3, curriculum integration is considered as a continuum, with levels representing its varying extent. These levels are applied to the medical curriculum with the aid of examples. Teacher-led integrations are distinguished from student-derived integrations, and the need for the teacher to plan activities that encourage the latter is emphasised. The concepts of horizontal and vertical integration are applied to the medical curriculum and the different organising themes to facilitate such integration presented.

Chapter 4 is devoted to a discussion, with examples, of integration practices in the medical curriculum. These practices are component-based, horizontal, vertical, problem-based, community-based and multiprofessional. The integration of the art and science of medicine is considered in relation to two trends that have developed in the curriculum: communication skills training and the introduction of medical ethics. Examples are drawn from the literature and from the author's personal experiences.

In Chapter 5, the advantages and disadvantages of an integrated medical curriculum are discussed. Advantages accrue to both the student and the teacher: to the former, relevance, understanding and retention; to the latter, collaboration, harmony and learning gains. The disadvantages of an integrated curriculum are more perceived than real, and are related to time and difficulty of implementation. The main concern is, however, an attitudinal one: a feeling of loss of territorial power when disciplinary boundaries become blurred.

In Chapter 6, the importance of assessment procedures that test the student's ability to form links among the content areas is stressed, as assessment determines the manner in which students learn. Examples of different types of items that test this ability are given and an institutional system for developing integrated test items is suggested. Some problems associated with an integrated system of assessment are discussed.

The evaluation of an integrated curriculum, whether it be new or a replacement of an existing programme, is considered in Chapter 7. A deficiency model of evaluation, which considers the context, inputs, processes and products of the programme, is proposed. The importance of both ongoing monitoring and summative evaluation for programme development is pointed out, as is the need for follow-up studies.

Chapter 8 is perhaps most significant for those who wish to plan and implement integrated curricula, as it identifies some of the pitfalls in implementing an integrated curriculum and suggests guidelines that would maximise the chances of success. These guidelines are developed from principles of learning and curriculum planning.

The final chapter describes and analyses four case studies of integrated courses or curricula with which the author was closely associated. The lessons learnt from each, as well as a comparison of the four, supplement the guidelines developed in the previous chapter.

It is the author's hope that the trend of integration of the medical curriculum, which is at last showing signs of gathering momentum, will spread to even the most traditional curricula and that this book will facilitate that spread.

Raja C Bandaranayake
January 2011

REFERENCES

1 Australian Medical Council. *Guidelines for the Assessment and Accreditation of Medical Schools*. Woden, ACT: Australian Medical Council; 1998.
2 World Federation for Medical Education. *Global Standards for Quality Improvement in Basic Medical Education*. Copenhagen: World Federation for Medical Education; 2003.
3 Liaison Committee on Medical Education. *Functions and Structure of a Medical School, Standards for Accreditation of Medical Education Programs Leading to the MD Degree*. Washington, DC: LCME; 2010.
4 General Medical Council. *Tomorrow's Doctors: outcomes and standards for undergraduate medical education*. London: General Medical Council; 2009.
5 Gulf Cooperation Council Medical Colleges Deans' Committee. Recommendations and guidelines on minimum standards for establishing

and accrediting medical schools in the Arabian Gulf countries (unpublished document), May 2001.

6 Proceedings of the First Asia Pacific Medical Education Conference. *Changing Paradigms*; 2003. Dec 3–5; Singapore.

About the author

Raja C Bandaranayake is a medical graduate of the University of Ceylon with a PhD in neuroanatomy from the University of London (Guy's Hospital Medical School). During a career in anatomy, he developed a keen interest in medical Education, obtaining a master's degree in this field from the University of Southern California. As an international consultant in medical education he has undertaken almost 100 consultations across some 30 countries, largely in curriculum, assessment and evaluation. Recently, he contributed to the development of international standards in basic medical education as a member of both the Task Force of the World Federation for Medical Education and the Core Group of the Institute for International Medical Education. He has published widely in the field of medical education. He now lives in retirement in Sydney, Australia, but continues to do consultative work.

Acknowledgements

The stimulus for my interest in medical education was created by the late Professor Senaka Bibile, Foundation Dean of the Faculty of Medicine and Dentistry, University of Ceylon, Peradeniya. His foresight in initiating a study group in this field as far back as 1962, viewed cynically by some at first, was largely responsible for the prominent place this medical school attained in the world of medical education in its early years. I acknowledge his lasting contribution to the school and to my career development.

I am indebted to that doyen of medical education, Emeritus Professor Stephen Abrahamson, of the University of Southern California School of Medicine in Los Angeles, who was my mentor in this field. I learnt much from him, not only in medical education, but also about how to help others to develop as educationists. My interest in the integrated curriculum commenced during my studentship under him, and he introduced me to many individuals who had similar interests. Words are inadequate to express the depth of my gratitude to him. I also thank him for contributing a Foreword to this book during his well-deserved retirement.

Many of the thoughts in this book resulted from my consultancies and study visits to medical schools in different parts of the world. While thanking international and national organisations, in particular the World Health Organization, for affording me the opportunities to make those visits, I am particularly grateful to the students, staff and administrators in those institutions for giving me their time and attention during the many discussions we had. It is impossible to name those institutions individually. My own postgraduate students and peers, particularly in the Medical Education Unit, Faculty of Medicine and Dentistry, University of Ceylon, Peradeniya; in the School of Medical Education, University of New South Wales, Sydney; and in the College of Medicine and Medical Sciences, Arabian Gulf University, Bahrain, contributed in no small measure to these thoughts, for which I am thankful.

Work on this book started many years ago but required the time and concentrated effort that only retirement after a busy working life could bring. During all those years the support of my wife, Chandrani, and my children, Rohan, Ruveni and Roshini, was indispensable. I thank them for their abiding patience.

Finally, I would like to thank my esteemed colleague Professor Ronald Harden of the University of Dundee for writing a second Foreword to this book despite his numerous commitments.

To my parents
Artin & Phoebe
from whom I inherited the love of teaching

CHAPTER 1

Integration and the medical curriculum

THE MEANING OF INTEGRATION

The term *integration* is used in so many walks of life that it has come to have several meanings. In the social context integration refers to the process by which two or more ethnic, racial or religious groups accept and live harmoniously with one another so that they contribute to the welfare of that society. In the political context integration refers to the process by which a group of nations comes together on issues of common interest and provision of mutual support while maintaining individual territorial rights. In psychology integration refers to the organisation of the constituent elements of the personality into a coordinated, harmonious whole. In mathematics integration refers to the operation of finding the integral of a function or equation, where an integer refers to a whole number as distinct from a fraction. To the theist integration means salvation of the soul, a state of eternal reality through 'oneness with the Almighty',[1] whoever that may be according to one's conviction. To the poet, the artist or the composer integration is the process of creation, by assimilating abstract concepts in the 'mind's eye', of a masterpiece that others can appreciate.

The many meanings of the term have the potential to create confusion, depending on the perspectives of the individuals involved in communication. The negative impact of such confusion in attempts at curriculum integration is highlighted in Chapter 8. Nevertheless, two common features of its varied usages are, first, a notion of bringing things together and, second, harmony in that union.

Webster's Encyclopedic Dictionary defines integration as 'combining or co-ordinating separate elements so as to provide a harmonious interrelated whole'.[2] This implies that parts exist that can be brought together into a whole. 'Whole' and 'part' in this sense are relative, in that a whole formed of certain parts could, in turn, be part of another whole. For example, an individual is part of a family (the whole) while the family is part of a community (a larger whole). In addition, the same part could contribute to several different wholes. In the same example, the same individual may also be a member (part) of an organisation (a different whole).

Integration is not merely a summation of different parts to make a whole. As Capehart aptly states, '[s]everal units do not add up to unity'.[3] The interrelationships among the units in the composite must also be included in the equation. In the example given, the individual members of a family do not make up a 'meaningful' family if their relationships to each other are ignored. Integration thus assumes the existence of parts within the composite that can be brought into relation with each other to make the composite more meaningful.

What do we understand by the word 'meaningful'? An object or event is meaningful to an individual to the extent that it fits with what that individual already knows or has experienced from the past. The perception of meaning, like learning, is an individual matter, in that what is meaningful for one may be less so for another. A little child does not immediately perceive meaning in a family that includes a new stepfather, as the latter was not part of the family earlier. His presence in the family creates dissonance in the child's perception of its family based on previous experience. The child is unable to integrate, in its own mind, the stepfather into its family.

The term meaningful as used earlier relates to concordance between the past and the present. It can also be used in another sense, whereby the present is related to the future. We derive meaning from an object or event if we can perceive the extent to which it coincides with our envisaged personal future. Each of us has some sort of notion about our future, either what it holds for us or what we would like it to be. The present experience has more meaning if it relates in some way to that perception of the future. In this sense the term meaningful is, perhaps, synonymous with relevance. Extending our example further, an older child may see more meaning in the presence of the stepfather if the latter's presence fits with the child's notion of its or its family's future. If it does, the child may come to accept the newcomer more easily.

The ability to integrate or integrative capacity, then, is related to one's experience of the past and perception of the future, both of which vary with maturity. Integrative capacity is at its maximum if the whole derived from the parts is consonant with one's experiences of the past and perceptions of the future.

Integration is both a verb and a noun. As a verb it is the act of bringing the parts of the whole together in meaningful relationships with one another. As a noun it is the state of unity that is achieved as a result of this act. It is a dynamic, not a static, state of equilibrium. An individual's experiences and perceptions change as the world around them changes. Thus one could never hope to achieve a complete or final state of integration. In most spheres of life, 'the integration of one century cannot be the integration of another century',[1] as knowledge grows and circumstances change. It is this very dynamic nature of integration that gives the zest for life and makes the individual strive for increasing levels of integration. A steady state would be monotonous. From an epistemological view-point, ultimate reality can never be achieved by mortal man. As he strives to get closer, it moves further, making the search an unending one.[4] He must, however, believe in the existence of a universe of truth that is susceptible to integration if he is to strive to achieve it.[5] If he does not, he has to be helped to believe in it by those who mould his life. The latter tend to look at reality from their respective perspectives, and unwittingly condition their disciples to adopt the same perspectives.

In his book *The Encapsulated Man*, Royce enumerates four epistemologies in man's search for ultimate reality: the rationalistic, intuitive, empirical and authoritarian approaches.[4] While each individual may use all four approaches, his primary dependence is on any one of them, based on his acculturation. The scientist tends to use the empirical approach predominantly, while the artist and the poet use the intuitive approach. To a large extent we all depend on the authoritarian approach, where those who have gone before us have documented their perceptions of reality. The blind acceptance of such authority, however, varies in degree among us, depending on the extent to which we are conditioned to question such authority. Royce contends that we only catch glimpses of reality through the perforations in the cocoon that encapsulates us, and that the scientist's view of reality may differ from the artist's, for example. As we become increasingly aware of other approaches to the truth, the integrations we make become increasingly complete.

The meaningful nature of an experience is related to the environment in which that experience takes place. Environment is both physical and psychological. Before he wrote his biographical novel, *The Torch*, on the life and times of Hippocrates,[6] Penfield visited the island of Cos where the Father of Modern Medicine practised and taught his profession to his disciples. Penfield placed himself in the physical environment in which the subject of his work lived in order to experience it himself. In his own words he 'breathed the air that Hippocrates breathed',[7] and in this intense state of meditation he, a renowned neuroscientist, saw a vision that tied together the threads of and provided the missing links for his story. One way in which he entered the psychological environment, which facilitated his integration of the facts of the life of Hippocrates, was to experience the actual physical environment that Hippocrates experienced. Penfield was able to break through his empirical and authoritarian cocoons and enter an intuitive cocoon, often associated with the poet, the artist or the cleric.

Penfield achieved integration by harmonising, in a meaningful way, his experiences of the past with those of the present, in relation to a pre-identified purpose. He thus maximised the conditions at his disposal to arrive at what was for him a more meaningful whole. In his search there would undoubtedly have been many questions unanswered, many discrepancies unaccounted for and many nagging doubts about the accuracy of what he saw in his mind's eye. That was what drove him to ever-increasing heights in his search for the truth, generating motivation for a challenging, yet unending, search. As Benor states, 'broadening the mental set to create patterns and thus enhance the flow of relevant associations is what integration is all about'.[8]

THE NATURE OF THE CURRICULUM

The curriculum has been defined as a series of planned activities that bring about learning in the students who are subjected to it. Undoubtedly, in the academic life of a student, much learning takes place from unplanned activities and events over which the curriculum planner has no control; and nor for that matter does the student have control over many of them. Such unplanned learning is of great significance, particularly in relation to the integration that takes place in the mind of the student. If what the student learns in the formal curriculum does not fit with incidental learning, dissonance results. If it contradicts, he has to make a choice or arrive at a compromise to overcome the dissonance. The importance of this to learning in medical school is discussed further in Chapter 3. In spite of the importance of unplanned learning experiences, the lack of control that the educationist has over them precludes their further consideration in issues of curriculum planning.

The curriculum is both a plan and a process. As a plan, it is usually documented and readily available for anyone to see. From such documents an idea may be obtained about its nature. As a process, it refers to the manner in which the plan is translated into action. The nature of the curriculum as a process can be determined by observing its implementation or through descriptions provided by the main players – namely, the students, faculty and administrators – after the event, based on their respective experiences. Often the plan and the process do not coincide, as the best intentions may not always be translated into appropriate actions.

An example from medical education illustrates this dichotomy between the curriculum on paper and the curriculum in action. The behavioural objectives movement ignited the world of medical education and spread through it like wildfire over the last three decades of the twentieth century. Spurred on by educational psychologists and medical educationists, medical teachers in many countries spent large amounts of time and effort, in the 1970s and 1980s, in compiling specific behavioural objectives, according to the criteria laid down by psychologists such as Mager.[9] Objectives so compiled were proudly displayed as the fruits of this labour. The energy expended by faculty was often so great, however, that once the chore was completed the product bore little relationship to the actual teaching. As a result the tomes of objectives so produced sat on bookshelves collecting dust, or in filing cabinets collecting mould. In one country teams of discipline specialists from the major medical schools spent several weeks compiling objectives in each discipline. This resulted in an impressive collection of books from which both students and teachers could have derived maximum benefit. The influence they had on the actual curriculum in practice, however, was marginal. Inquiry about them in one medical school produced expressions of surprise at their existence. Some teachers were not even aware of such a resource, let alone making use of them.

The curriculum is a system of component parts that are related to each other structurally and functionally.[10] As with any system each component must function properly if the system is to work. A change affecting one component would have repercussions on the entire system. If steps are not taken to effect corresponding changes in the others, the functioning of the system as a whole is affected. For example, if teaching methods change without corresponding changes in methods of assessment, it is unlikely that the change in teaching method would have the desired effects. The realisation of this issue is of critical importance for successful integration, and is discussed in depth in Chapter 6.

A curriculum consists of a series of planned educational experiences with a definite purpose in mind. Each learning experience has to take into consideration the experiences that preceded it, those that accompany it and those that are to follow it. A collection of learning experiences, each of which by itself is a good experience, does not make a good curriculum if the relationships among the learning experiences are ignored.

To be effective, new learning, which is built on existing learning, must be related to past learning. Planned and unplanned learning experiences differ from each other in that lack of control over the latter results in unrelated experiences without a logical sequence. On the other hand, planned educational experiences are arranged in a sequence that facilitates the progression of the learner from one segment of learning to the next. The sequence has some internal logic about it, such as increasing levels of competence in a field, where earlier units are pre-requisite to subsequent units. As the learner sees the relationships between the new learning and the old, the latter is reinforced and the former integrated into the learner's knowledge or skill base. When two learning units are concurrent the extent to which they complement each other depends on their relatedness to each other. When the learner recognises these relationships the learning of each is reinforced by the other and is most effective.

The spiral curriculum is one in which concepts learnt in previous segments of the curriculum are brought back repeatedly in later segments and at increasing levels of complexity. The concepts learnt earlier are reinforced and they facilitate the integration of their more complex aspects introduced later. A typical example of this is seen in some problem-centred curricula where 'iterative exposure to the sciences at progressively more complex levels can contribute to cumulative learning'.[11] Retention of learning is most effective when reinforced across different segments and phases of a curriculum.

INTEGRATION IN RELATION TO THE CURRICULUM

In a general sense education is preparation for life. The more educated a person is the richer that person's life is. Education creates in the individual an awareness of the world around him, of the opportunities to find his niche in that world and of his potential to avail himself of those opportunities. The challenge involved in striving to achieve the maximum of one's potential is what gives richness to life. This does not mean that the uneducated are not content with life. Contentment is determined by the extent of the discrepancy between what the individual perceives as attainable and what he actually attains. One could say that the less educated a person is the less awareness he has of what is attainable, and the smaller the discrepancy. The educated person may have a higher level of discontent if he is unable to achieve what he perceives as attainable. Nevertheless, unless the discrepancy is so great as to create frustration, the struggle for achievement gives purpose and meaning to life, adding to its richness.

Professional education is preparation for a life of service to society in a given field of human endeavour. The purpose of professional school is to develop in the future practitioner those abilities prerequisite to the provision of professional service. Self-directed learning and problem solving are two skills that would equip the future practitioner for facing the uncertainties of professional life. The ability to integrate learning throughout professional life with previous learning, as well as with the realities of the world around him, is another skill that would be invaluable to the continuing learner and practitioner.

Integration of learning takes place in the mind of the learner. Like learning, it is an individual activity as learners differ in what they find meaningful. We differ in our past experiences, our perceptions of the world around us and our expectations for the future. As Dressel repeatedly emphasises, the curriculum should try to develop individuals who integrate for themselves, rather than those who accept the integrations made by others.[12] The learner who is exposed to an integrated unit within the curriculum may derive meaning from it by relating it to past experience and future expectations without having undergone the mental exercise of identifying those relationships himself.

The teacher has an important role to play in developing integrating learners. First, the teacher acts as a role model to the learners by demonstrating integrative behaviour and exposing the latter to integrations made by others. Second, the teacher facilitates integrating activity undertaken by the learners by creating the conditions for learning that are conducive to such activity. If the teacher depends exclusively on the first type of activity, the more passive learners, who are accustomed to accepting authority, will not question the former's integrations in their attempts to derive as much meaning as possible from them. On the other hand, the teacher who engages exclusively in the second type of activity may leave the less creative learners without a model on which to base their integrating task. The challenge to the teacher is, therefore, to arrive at a delicate balance between these two extremes of integrated and integrating experiences.

Whether a learner, in spite of the teacher's intentions, engages in integrating activity depends on a number of factors related to the learner's motivation, knowledge base and awareness of the potential for integration. Motivation is enhanced when the relevance of integration to the perceived goal is seen by the learner. Short-term goals that act as a driving force include the common immediate concern for learners that they succeed in examinations. The relationship between motivation for integrating behaviour and the nature of examinations is discussed further in Chapter 6. The more important, long-term goals are related to the professional's future practice. The relevance of integration to professional work is perceived by learners when they see experienced professionals demonstrate integrating behaviour in their practice. This requires such professionals who interact with learners to consciously demystify their behaviours when engaged in the practice of their profession concurrently with teaching. Pattern recognition engaged in by the experienced clinician, for example, is mystifying to the novice, who may not perceive the mental integrations achieved by the former in arriving at a diagnosis.

Undoubtedly, an adequate knowledge base is prerequisite for integrating behaviour to occur. This may be taken to imply that mastery of the parts that comprise a whole must precede integration. However, learning does not necessarily progress from parts to whole. The whole may be presented first, with the learners encouraged to analyse it and break it up into its constituent parts. Although the process of integration itself is a synthetic mental activity, an analytical approach where the whole is dissected into its constituent parts also helps the learner perceive the relationships among the constituent parts, just as much as a technician may disassemble a complex machine into its component parts before learning to reassemble it. Integrated learning units in a curriculum may thus be arranged in a simple to complex sequence, as is common in the more conventional curricula that adopt a 'building blocks' approach; or around problems that require analysis before synthesis, such as in problem-centred curricula.

Self-awareness of the learner's potential for integrating activity is developed through frequent exposure to situations that require the learner to engage in such activity. Formative assessments are usually not associated with integrating activity, as they are diagnostic in nature, requiring the learner to demonstrate mastery of the parts, rather than the whole. Summative assessment, on the other hand, should focus on the whole, and the ability of the learner to relate the mastered parts to this whole. The nature of such assessment is discussed in Chapter 6.

Reality is the substrate for integration, as reality is meaningful. The power of integrations made in daily life is derived from the reality of life experiences. Planned educational experiences in the real world are more conducive to integrated learning than those that are organised in the artificial world of the classroom. However, we cannot stage all learning experiences, or each in its entirety, in the unpredictable real world of future practice. The curriculum planner can certainly be expected, however, to arrange as many of the experiences as possible in situations that mimic the real world of future practice as closely as possible. Ker *et al.* demonstrated the power of learning experiences organised in realistic and safe simulated clinical settings for second-year medical and nursing students.[13] Learning that takes place in an environment that resembles as closely as possible that in which the learner applies the learning is seen as meaningful and, hence, is more likely to be integrated.[14]

Krathwohl points out that effective integration is more easily achieved if the drive for integration is related to the learner's felt need.[15] It was pointed out above that the motivation for integration is increased if the learner perceives its relationship to the long-term goals of professional practice. Often the learner may not be immediately aware of the relevance of a unit of learning, or of the integration of learning within that unit, to future professional practice. The unit then does not fall within the ambit of the learner's felt needs. The teacher who encourages integrating behaviour in the learner would not merely state that the unit is relevant to future practice but also would take steps to relate present learning to future practice.

Professional practice requires the learner in professional school to develop those competencies that have been identified as prerequisite to practice. Curricula that are based on competencies of professional practice focus on the functions expected of the graduate, thereby enhancing the relationship between the latter's educational experience and eventual work. Educational objectives for such curricula are derived from the real world of professional practice by examining the roles of the professional in different practice settings. Competencies on which such curricula are based are derived from needs that may arise from several sources, of which the learner is only one. The needs of the employer, the profession, the professional school and the community also determine the competencies for the professional curriculum.

A potential danger of a competency-based curriculum is the disintegrative nature of the analytical process involved in deriving educational objectives from professional competencies. Some writers even differentiate among subject-centred, integrated and competency-based curricular models[16] as though they are mutually exclusive. It may be argued that even the differentiation between subject-centred and integrated curricula is artificial. A curriculum may be integrated to different degrees, as part and whole in relation to a curriculum are relative. Thus, rather than dichotomise integrated and non-integrated curricula, it is preferable, from both philosophical and practical points of view, to view curricular integration on a continuum. One curriculum may be more integrated than another depending on the basis of integration – namely, the nature of the whole. Even a subject-centred curriculum may manifest a considerable degree of integration within each subject. Characterising problem-based curricula as 'fully integrated' or subject-centred curricula as devoid of any integration is errone-ous,[17] as total integration cannot be achieved, nor can integration be completely avoided. Admittedly, a curriculum that transcends the artificial boundaries laid down by subjects or disciplines has integrative capabilities at a higher level than a subject-centred one, as the real-life situations that the professional is likely to encounter in practice do not respect disciplines. From a practical point of view the curriculum developer should encourage increasing degrees of integration without denying, or diminishing the value of, integrations that inevitably occur in any given curriculum.

Differentiating competency-based curricula from integrated curricula is illogical as the former are characterised by a particular way of deriving content – namely, from an analysis of competencies – and the latter, by the manner in which this content is organised. The two are not mutually exclusive. This dis-tinction is amplified in Chapter 3. Even though content may be derived from an analytical process, it may subsequently be synthesised, for teaching purposes, to form meaningful wholes.

The manner in which curricular units are organised and sequenced is an important determiner of the nature of curricular integration. For practical rea-sons, curricular content is necessarily packaged into smaller units. Traditionally, units represent the disciplines of which the content of the curriculum is com-prised. Integrated curricula attempt to reorganise the content into units or packages that are more meaningful to the learner in that they are closer to the entities that the professional is likely to experience in practice than the artificial categories represented by the disciplines. Meaningful re-organisation is based on certain themes or threads, discussed later in Chapter 3.

Sequencing is the manner in which the curricular units are arranged on the temporal axis. It is in part determined by the prerequisites that the learner must master before proceeding to a given unit. If learning experiences are to have a cumulative effect they must be so organised as to reinforce each other. Well-planned educational experiences have a sequential relationship so that each new experience is related to past experiences and has the potential to relate to future experiences.[18] The dual nature of meaningful integrations, in relation to previous learning as well as to future application, was pointed out earlier. To enhance integrated learning, curricular units must be so sequenced that new units are related to previous units as well as to future application. In addition concurrent units should reinforce one another by the relationships among them being brought to the attention of the learner or through opportunities provided for the learner to relate them to one another at the time they are being imple-mented. The inter-relationships among courses are one of the keys to curricular integration.

In summary, then, a curriculum is integrated to the extent that it encourages learners to undertake integrative activity on their own, but provides models to facilitate their doing so; caters to the needs of the learners while assisting them to identify these needs; packages the content within it into units that are closer to the entities that the learner is likely to encounter in practice; arranges these units in a sequence that enables them to relate their learning to previous learning; recreates in the learner's mind at least, if not in reality, the actual environment in which the learner would apply that learning; and brings into focus the application of that learning in future units and in professional practice. While no curriculum plan could hope to achieve all these attributes in entirety, the aim of the body responsible for curriculum planning should be to achieve them to the maximum level possible given the particular circumstances of the situation.

KEY POINTS

- Integration is combining separate elements into a meaningful whole.
- Integrative capacity is related to previous experience (meaningfulness) and perceived future (relevance).
- Both meaningfulness and relevance of an experience are related to the physiological and psychological environment in which that experience takes place.
- The curriculum is a system of components related to one another.
- The curriculum on paper may not match the curriculum in practice.
- The skilled professional integrates new learning with previous learning throughout their professional life.
- The teacher's role is to develop learners who are able to integrate for themselves.
- Motivation and a knowledge base are a prerequisite for developing integrating learners.

REFERENCES

1 Organ T. The philosophical basis of integration. In: Henry NB, editor. *The Integration of Educational Experiences*, 57th Yearbook of the National Society for the Study of Education, Part III. Chicago, IL: University of Chicago Press; 1958, Chapter II, pp. 26–42.

2 *Webster's Encyclopedic Dictionary*, New York, NY: Lexicon; 1989.

3 Capehart BE. Illustrative courses and programs in selected secondary schools. In: Henry NB, editor. *The Integration of Educational Experiences*, op. cit., Chapter X, pp. 194–217.

4 Royce JR. *The Encapsulated Man*. Princeton, NJ: Von Nostrand; 1964. pp. 11–19.

5 Mayhew LB. Illustrative courses and programs in colleges and universities. In: Henry NB, editor. *The Integration of Educational Experiences*, op. cit., Chapter XI, pp. 218–48.

6 Penfield WG. *The Torch*. Boston, MA: Little, Brown & Co.; 1960.

7 Penfield WG. From hippocratic facts to fiction. *Clin Neurosurg.* 1956; 4: 11–20.

8 Benor DE. Interdisciplinary integration in medical education: theory and method. *Med Educ.* 1982; **16**: 355–61.

9 Mager RF. *Preparing Instructional Objectives.* Palo Alto, CA: Fearon; 1962.

10 Rotem A, Bandaranayake R. How to plan and conduct programme evaluation. *Med Teach.* 1983; **5**: 127–31.

11 Engel CE, Clarke RM. Medical education with a difference. *PLET.* 1979; **16**: 72–87.

12 Dressel PL. The meaning and significance of integration. In: Henry NB, editor. *The Integration of Educational Experiences,* op. cit., Chapter I, pp. 3–25.

13 Ker J, Mole L, Bradley P. Early introduction to interprofessional learning: a simulated ward environment. *Med Educ.* 2003; **37**: 248–55.

14 Bandaranayake R. The integrated medical curriculum. In: Bandaranayake R, editor. *Trends in Curricula.* Sydney: University of New South Wales Press; 1979. pp. 1–10.

15 Krathwohl DR. The psychological bases for integration. In: Henry NB, editor. *The Integration of Educational Experiences,* op. cit., Chapter III, pp. 43–65.

16 McGaghie WC, Miller GE, Sajid AW, *et al.* Competency-based curriculum development in medical education: an introduction. *Public Health Pap.* 1978; **68**: 11–91.

17 Heylings DJ. Anatomy 1999–2000: the curriculum, who teaches it and how? *Med Educ.* 2002; **36**: 702–10.

18 Bloom BS. Ideas, problems and methods of inquiry. In: Henry NB, editor. *The Integration of Educational Experiences,* op. cit., Chapter V, pp. 84–104.

CHAPTER 2

The history of the integrated medical curriculum

THE GROWTH OF THE SPECIALITIES

The earliest known attempt at integrated medical teaching could be said to have taken place under the celebrated plane tree on the island of Cos in the Aegean Sea, where Hippocrates taught his disciples the foundations of modern medicine. Medical knowledge was so circumscribed at the time, and the skills of medicine so limited, that the need to package the content into smaller units did not exist. Hippocrates was able not only to integrate this knowledge and impart it to his disciples but also to combine the skill and the art of medical practice, as was evidenced by the enunciation of his famous Oath.

The exponential increase in medical knowledge and the concomitant development of technical skills since that time resulted in the growth of the specialities, and subsequently of the sub-specialities, as we know them. As medical education began to be institutionalised each major speciality carved out for itself an area of content with responsibility for teaching that content decentralised in a few self-contained institutional units called departments. As the body of knowledge and skills related to each speciality grew, increasing divisions within each department resulted in a proliferation of departments and sub-departments, each with a considerable degree of autonomy in relation to planning and implementing the curriculum. For example, anatomy and physiology, including histology, were at one time the responsibility of a single department, from which anatomy separated first, followed by histology, which established itself either as a separate department or a sub-department within anatomy. Subsequently, pharmacology and biochemistry separated from physiology. Thus from one department grew five, each with its own body of knowledge, jealously guarded by its exponents, and continuing to grow in size. If one were to closely examine a department of physiology in a larger university today, one would in fact find not just a unitary department but several sub-departments within it, related to such sub-specialities as neurophysiology, cardiovascular physiology and renal physiology. The rapid growth of sub-specialities is exemplified by the fact that, in 1965, Child identified 18 subdivisions of surgery (excluding anaesthesia),[1] while Lord, in 1992, identified 31 sections or subdivisions of surgery that were either proposed or formed within the Royal Australasian College of Surgeons between the years 1950 and 1990.[2]

Disciplines evolve over a long period of time and are identified by boundaries that at times may be indistinct. The specialist, identified with a particular discipline, tends to 'discipline' those who come into contact with him. The longer the discipline survives the more firmly is it rooted and the more it resists encroachment by, or merging with, other disciplines.[3] It is not unusual, however, for a branch of the original fundamental discipline to align itself with an applied component of professional education and form a separate sub-department of either the fundamental or the applied discipline. The birth of hybrid departments such as clinical physiology may be attributed to this merging of departments at the interface between them in an attempt to relate basic to applied aspects. While such hybrids contribute to integration of subject areas their potential danger lies in the effect they have on the original departments from which they branched. It is easy for a department of physiology, for example, to delegate applied aspects of its content to the hybrid and continue to teach the fundamental discipline as a subject in its own right, without relating it to application.

Each discipline develops its own logical sequence, which is intrinsic to it.[4] As the discipline grows, this sequence becomes part of its tradition, and attempts to rearrange it are thwarted by its proponents. Allegiance to the discipline is so strong that it often supersedes the ultimate aim of the curriculum, and the integrity of the discipline itself, rather than of the profession of which it forms part, becomes the focus. As institutions grow in size and complexity, departments within each do likewise, adding strength to the individual parts and splintering the complex into increasingly smaller fragments. Each smaller unit follows the same trend as its parent. The result is a conglomerate of complex departments that comprise the medical school of today. Dressel argues that 'compartmentalisation and specialisation are not solely the result of increasing knowledge, but also of the increasing size and complexity of educational institutions'.[5]

The growth of disciplines and departments in medical school is a self-augmenting process: increase in knowledge creates a discipline, which identifies itself within a separate department, which in turn creates more knowledge.

The tremendous advances of scientific knowledge in medicine are directly attributable to the growth of the specialities. As with scotomatous vision, specialists probe deeper into the limited area of their specialities, they uncover more and more scientific 'truth', which adds to the body of knowledge in their respective disciplines. In American medical education the oft-quoted Flexner Report[6] was a landmark in the development of the scientific foundation of medicine. Mayhew points out that in the medieval and early American university, religion was a focal point around which integration of the curriculum occurred.[7] American medical education, however, was largely outside the ambit of the liberal arts college and the professional university until Flexner's recommendations were implemented. Concern for the proliferation of substandard medical schools without the academic environment of the university was the stimulus of the Report, which advocated the development of the sciences basic to medicine. The incorporation of the medical school into the university gave professional training in medicine academic respectability, away from the trade school mentality it was rapidly developing. The time was ripe for the unbridled growth of the science of medicine, with an inevitable increase in the length and diversification of the curriculum. Segmentation of the curriculum, both vertically, into the premedical, preclinical and clinical phases as we know them today, and horizontally, into the familiar subjects within each phase, was but a step away.

Christie attributes to the Flexner Report in North America, to the Haldane and Goodenough reports in England and to the Debres Report in France the encouragement of full-time faculty appointments in medicine.[8] Attached to their respective departments faculty members immersed themselves in a narrow area of interest and developed expertise within it, often knowing as much of the other disciplines that impinged on this narrow area as even faculty members in those other disciplines. Research did not recognise boundaries between disciplines as long as the latter contributed to a solution of the problem at hand. But the narrowness of the area of interest precluded a significant multidisciplinary approach to teaching by the individual specialist. Willingness to transcend disciplinary boundaries in research did not carry over to teaching. Each discipline continued to be taught within the related department according to a logical organisation that was intrinsic to the discipline. Gross anatomy, for example, was sequenced on a body-regions basis, while physiology was on an organ-systems basis. In time, the sequence became traditional to the discipline. While this intrinsically logical sequence resulted in intradisciplinary integration, inter-relationships among the disciplines became more and more a rarity.

In due course, as knowledge advanced and the discipline fragmented further, the growth of the sub-specialities jeopardised even intradisciplinary integration. The growth of the specialities and sub-specialities resulted in each being taught as a discipline in its own right, with scant respect for the purpose for which it was taught to the medical student. Inevitably, the cry for relevance began to be heard in the corridors of medical education.

The 1960s was a period of turbulence in higher education in America, followed closely by the rest of the developed world. The fortuitous and synchronous merging of several incidents was responsible for this agitation in academia. Russia's early successes in the space race, the desegregation policy in schools, violence on campuses and a general lack of direction and purpose in higher education triggered student unrest, which gradually swelled into open revolt. Medical education, conservative as it always was, and often isolated from the rest of the university, was hardly affected by these early rumblings. Another development, however, was beginning to affect the nature of medical education. Concern over the unbridled growth of the curriculum, often associated with poor-quality teaching, had triggered a closer look at the nature of education imparted to the medical student by an overworked and often uncaring faculty.

The Project in Medical Education, at the State University of New York in Buffalo, was a happy union of education and medicine that gave birth to the discipline of medical education. The story of this movement, starting as a series of seminars in medical education and spreading to all corners of the globe, is vividly related by Miller.[9] One outcome of this movement was the realisation that medical school teachers, recruited on the basis of their academic standing in the profession, were generally inadequately prepared to undertake the task of educating the future professional. They needed to acquire pedagogic skills if they were to be entrusted with this serious task. The realisation that attention had to be paid to *what* was taught in addition to *how* it was taught was not long in coming. Enmeshed in the former was the issue of relevance. The cry for relevance in medical education was gathering momentum.

THE RISE OF THE INTEGRATED MEDICAL CURRICULUM

The fragmentation of the curriculum and the preoccupation of the subject matter specialist with his discipline had resulted in a centrifugal curriculum, at the centre of which was the student with her needs. Pulled in all directions by the demands made by each discipline, and buffeted by the varying pressures exerted by each at different times, the student succumbed to each force as and when it was exerted. Her education, too, became fragmented and the demands made by each speciality became so great that she hardly had time to assimilate the requirements of each, let alone study the relationships among them. As each department continued to demand her attention and time increasingly, she began to question the purpose of the voluminous content she was exposed to. Dissatisfaction was spreading among the usually docile medical student body as well.

Medical schools responded to these pressures in different ways. In the United States, influenced by the graduate nature of medical education, the training of the physician became increasingly focused on the specialist. In many medical schools a significant slice of the curriculum was designated elective to train the student in the chosen speciality while still in medical school. The resulting dearth of generalists in the American scene, and the reintroduction of family medicine as a speciality, is another story. On the other hand, specialist training was not considered the end product of undergraduate medical education in the United Kingdom and in those countries that inherited its system of medical education.

A six-year tertiary education was an expensive undertaking and the longest period of training prior to independent practice among the professions. Thus increasing the length of the undergraduate curriculum to accommodate the burgeoning content was not a viable option. In fact many schools shortened the curriculum in an effort to reduce costs and increase the years of productive service. Maintaining the length of the curriculum and increasing its content resulted in a crowded timetable with an increase in the more efficient but less effective didactic methods of teaching. Students had little time left to engage in reflective thinking on what they were learning. The detrimental effects of the accelerated medical curriculum in some American medical schools did not take long to manifest themselves in the students who were the victims of these experiments, and many of these curricula reverted to their former duration.

One of the most salutary effects of these developments in medical education was the opportunity it provided faculty members to rethink the way medical education was organised since the time of Flexner. Medical knowledge had grown to such an extent since that it undoubtedly had to be packaged in some form before it could be presented to the student. In isolated instances faculty members were beginning to ask whether this knowledge could be packaged in a way that was more conducive to its learning by the student than the divisions that through tradition had become so established in the medical curriculum. Consideration of the student and her needs as the centre of the curriculum marked the beginning of attempts to create a centripetal curriculum from one that had increasingly become centrifugal. A search for organising themes around which the packaging could occur led to the identification of the body organ systems as one common theme to all those disciplines that had blossomed in the post-Flexnerian era. The earliest school to consider such an organisation, as far back as 1952, was Western Reserve Medical School in Cleveland, Ohio.[10] Cross-disciplinary themes were considered desirable in the attempt to curb the autonomy of departments, which militated against a centripetal curriculum. Taking a leaf out of the book of secondary education, the medical school was sowing the seeds of integration in its curriculum.

More than two decades later the search for other integrating themes in medical education was still in progress. Educational concepts of learning through inquiry, discovery and problem solving, championed by educational psychologists such as Bruner[11], had already been sparingly applied in the elementary and secondary school. The pioneering curriculum at McMaster University's School of Medicine, established in 1968, adapted these concepts and practices to the medical curriculum.[12] Clinical problems were the organising theme around which the content of the medical curriculum was integrated. The recognition that undergraduate medical education was but a mere phase in a lifetime of professional learning led to the realisation of the importance to the future professional of a way to knowledge rather than knowledge itself. The skills of self-directed learning, of problem solving and of integrating one's learning were the foundation on which the curriculum in this and similar schools was built, not on a thick layer of the sciences basic to medicine. Knowledge for use rather than for its own sake was the key and its use was seen as solving problems that the future professional would encounter in every facet of her professional life. Integration in medical education had penetrated the psychological environment of the learner.

The invasion of the physical environment of the future professional remained. Until now the lecture theatre, the laboratory and the hospital had been the hallowed precincts of training for the profession. The increasing complexity of the teaching hospital had, in most instances, made it a tertiary care hospital. This was not, however, the environment in which the neophyte would apply the learning she had acquired in medical school. The importance of exposing the medical student to the community and its primary care facilities became increasingly recognised, just as community medicine gained prominence, at least in terms of curricular time if not in prestige. As community-based learning experiences were incorporated into the curriculum the monopoly that the teaching hospital held on the clinical phase of training was broken. To this day, however, the hospital continues to dominate the clinical training of the student, even though economic factors have influenced the gradual move of the clinical learning environment away from the tertiary care hospital to primary and secondary care venues in more recent years.

One other barrier remained to be broken if Hippocrates was to be revisited; namely, the integration of the science and the art of medicine.

INTEGRATION OF THE HUMANITIES WITH MEDICINE

The union of medicine with science had provided the foundation on which the rational practice of medicine was based, under the influence of visionaries such as Abraham Flexner. The manner in which the medical curriculum had developed – and develop it did in leaps and bounds – was so biased in the assumption that the sciences were the only foundation of clinical medicine that the art of medicine had long been forgotten. The disease, rather than the patient with the disease, became the focal point of both clinical practice and, consequently, the curriculum. As enormous strides in medical research resulted in the discovery of new diseases and their pathogenesis, and of sophisticated ways of investigating and managing disease conditions, the patient and his problem were often forgotten. Just as the disciplines in the medical curriculum had developed centrifugally, away from the student, so did medical practice from the patient. The disease-oriented curriculum had made it extremely difficult for the art of medicine to find its rightful place in the education of the future doctor. As Odegaard states in his thoughtful book *Dear Doctor: A Personal Letter to a Physician,*

> The entry of physicians into the university for professional education in the biosciences of the Flexnerian curriculum has exposed them to the attitudes and ideas associated with the scientific culture . . . [but they] have absorbed from their immediate intellectual environment . . .. a pejorative attitude toward representatives of the humanistic and social culture and their scholarly endeavours.[13]

Abraham Flexner had already foreseen this possibility when he published his report urging the development of the sciences basic to medicine. He predicted that the social role of the physician would expand once the scientific training was firmly established. It was several decades after Flexner, however, that those responsible for medical education came to realise that the rapid advances in medical science and technology were fast overtaking the humanistic side of medicine.[14]

Several factors contributed to the growth of the social and behavioural sciences in the medical curriculum. Medical litigation was on the rise and doctors were increasingly being held responsible for their actions and consequences. Concomitantly, the cost of medical insurance was rising and, as Harless *et al.* observed, physicians were prepared to withhold services from the public to thwart this rise.[15] The doctor–patient relationship was being gradually eroded, and the relative inadequacy of the former's communication ability was to a large extent responsible for this deteriorating state of affairs. Medical educators were increasingly recognising the need to correct the imbalance between the disease-oriented and patient-oriented curriculum.

Two strategies were adopted to steer the curriculum towards the art of medicine. The introduction of a separate behavioural sciences stream saw several types of courses being incorporated in the curriculum for a wide variety of purposes. Behavioural scientists, often unsure of the specific needs of the physician, selected content without proper use of criteria related to purpose. Thus they were unable to impress upon the student the importance of what they were teaching, and the student often regarded these subjects as 'soft'. The other strategy was to integrate behavioural science content into existing subjects. Unaccustomed as they were to teaching such content, due to the impersonal scientific tradition inculcated in them in medical school, faculty members were uneasy about such integration. Many medical schools employed clinical psychologists to undertake such teaching in conjunction with a medical specialist. However, the student who saw the practising clinician as his role model was more impressed by the latter demonstrating the humanistic side of medicine in his practice.

Over the last three decades the medical curriculum has shown a definite stream of behavioural science in its curriculum. It still suffers from a lack of clarity of purpose and from the reluctance of the clinician to compromise the science of medicine with its art in his teaching, even though he has realised the need for doing so in practice. Medical ethics courses have sprung up in many medical schools, most often as separate entities.[16,17] Yet the more effective ones are those that, integrated into existing courses, require the students to examine the ethical dilemmas that the physician faces in his daily practice. Slowly but surely the art of medicine is finding its rightful place in the medical curriculum.

KEY POINTS

- The exponential growth of knowledge resulted in its compartmentalisation into disciplines and sub-disciplines.
- Each discipline developed an expanding body of knowledge and an intrinsic logical sequence.
- Unbridled growth of the content in each discipline and its inclusion in the curriculum resulted in concerns about relevance.
- In looking for organising themes for rearranging content in other ways, curriculum planners considered body organ systems and later clinical problems.
- Learning in community settings gained prominence with the realisation that the community was a major practising environment of the future professional.
- Integration of the art and science of medicine came about to counter the undue emphasis placed on the disease rather than the patient with the disease.

REFERENCES

1 Child CG. General surgery, surgical specialties and medical education. *J Med Educ.* 1965; **40**: 703–11.

2 Lord RS. The fragmentation of general surgery. *Aust N Z J Surg.* 1992; **62**: 175–80.

3 Eye GG. As far as the Eye can see: educational shackle-breakers. *J Educ Res.* 1975; **68**: 202–7.

4 Capehart BE. Illustrative courses and programs in selected secondary schools. In: Henry NB, editor. *The Integration of Educational Experiences*, 57th Yearbook of the National Society for the Study of Education, Part III, Chicago, IL: University of Chicago Press, 1958, Chapter X, pp. 194–217.

5 Dressel PL. Integration: an expanding concept. In: Henry NB, editor. *The Integration of Educational Experiences*, op. cit., Chapter XII, pp. 251–63.

6 Flexner A. Medical Education in the United States and Canada: A report to the Carnegie Foundation for the Advancement of Teaching. *Bulletin Number 4*, Boston, MA: Merrymount; 1910.

7 Mayhew LB. Illustrative courses and programs in colleges and universities. In: Henry NB, editor. *The Integration of Educational Experiences*, op. cit., Chapter XI, pp. 218–48.

8 Christie RV. Trends in medical education. *J Med Educ.* 1963; **38**: 662–6.

9 Miller GE. *Educating Medical Teachers*. Cambridge, MA: Harvard University Press. 1980.

10 Ham TH. Medical education at Western Reserve University. A progress report for the sixteen years, 1946–1962. *N Engl J Med* 1962; **267**: 868–74, 916–23.

11 Bruner JS. *The Process of Education*. New York: Vintage Books; 1963, Chapter 2, pp. 20–1.

12 Neufeld VR, Barrows HS. The 'McMaster Philosophy': an approach to medical education. *J Med Educ.* 1974; **49**: 1040–50.

13 Odegaard CE. *Dear Doctor: a personal letter to a physician.* Memorial Park, CA: Henry J Kaiser Family Foundation; 1986.

14 Gwee M. The introduction of social and behavioural sciences into the medical curriculum. In: Bandaranayake R, editor. *Trends in Curricula.* Sydney: University of New South Wales Press; 1979. p. 11.

15 Harless WG, Farr NA, Zier MA, *et al.* MERIT – an application of CASE. In: DeLand EC, editor. *Information Technology in Health Science Education.* New York, NY: Plenum Press; 1978. pp. 565–9.

16 Puthucheary SD. A curriculum in medical ethics and medical humanities. *Med J Malaysia.* 1980; **35**: 86–95.

17 Al-Mahroos F, Bandaranayake R. Teaching medical ethics in medical schools (Editorial). *Ann Saudi Med.* 2003; **23**: 1–5.

CHAPTER 3

Levels and types of integration in the medical curriculum

THE EXTENT OF INTEGRATION

Curricular integration, as pointed out in Chapter 1, is relative in nature in that the whole in one context can be part of a larger whole. Integration may involve, at one extreme, a single lesson, and at the other, the entire curriculum. In fact the level of integration may be extended even further, so that the undergraduate curriculum may be integrated with postgraduate and continuing education. Dressel points out that the 'whole' may be the individual, society, curriculum or even all knowledge.[1] As integration can take place even within the smallest segment of the curriculum, it must follow that every curriculum is integrated to some extent. It would be hard to imagine a teacher who does not attempt to integrate a single lesson. The dichotomy often implied in the literature between 'integrated' and 'traditional' curricula is, therefore, erroneous.

Often contrasted with the integrated curriculum is the discipline-oriented curriculum. Such a contrast carries the notion that a discipline-oriented curriculum cannot be integrated, when in the overwhelming majority of medical schools the department is the unit responsible for teaching, and the curriculum is structured around the disciplines. It would be far more profitable to think in terms of a continuum of integration. While recognising that all curricula have some inherent degree of integration, each may be placed at some point on the continuum based on parameters indicating the degree of integration. If integrated learning is considered desirable, and an integrated curriculum facilitates this, the aim should be to increase the degree of integration in the curriculum. Such an aim is much more likely to appeal to conservative medical faculty members than one that envisages a radical change in the fabric of the organisation by dismantling existing departments.

One of the most significant ways of achieving integration within a curriculum is through correlation of its component elements. This has its roots in the basic definition of integration, where summation of components is not, by itself, considered adequate for integration to occur. Integration implies an increase in the extent to which the whole created from summation is meaningful to the learner.

In terms of the curriculum, for the whole to be more meaningful the parts must be related to each other. Therein is the importance of correlation. Obvious as this may sound one is surprised at the lack of understanding displayed by many medical school teachers of this basic prerequisite for effective integration. Many curricula are labelled integrated just because they have in some way managed to combine different components. Abrahamson refers to this practice as 'integration by staple'.[2] As Dressel points out, correlation of independent subjects is different from the fusion of previously separate subjects.[1] In some instances such fusion is attempted by faculty members from different disciplines undertaking joint teaching sessions (team teaching). In others fusion is attempted by synchronising the teaching of the same content area by different disciplines. While these may all contribute to integration they do not necessarily guarantee that integrated learning is facilitated, simply because they do not ensure that the relationships among subjects are articulated.

An experience in a medical school demonstrated this confusion between fusion and integration clearly. One of the cornerstones on which the philosophy of this relatively young curriculum was built was integration. While some degree of integration was apparent in the earlier years this had been gradually eroded with time, ostensibly because of the logistic difficulties experienced in attempts at team teaching in the preclinical phase of the curriculum and at synchronisation in the clinical phase. The author was invited to advise the school as to how the original practices could be resurrected, given the present problems that the school faced. It soon became obvious that the erosion of integration in the curriculum had occurred simply because integration was equated, on the one hand, with team teaching and, on the other, with synchronisation. When it was pointed out that, while both of these practices could contribute to integration, neither was essential, and that emphasising relationships among the subjects was more important than either, the path to facilitating integration became clearer and more acceptable to the faculty. Preclinical teachers were able to develop a synchronised programme based on body organ systems and clinical teachers were able to develop a series of team-teaching activities. At the heart of both these efforts, however, were the correlations that were highlighted among the different subjects, which were the key to effective integration.

Curricula that are based on sequential learning, such as in medicine, require organisation of content into an appropriate sequence. While reorganisation of content may facilitate integration, this does not of itself ensure it. A strategy adopted by many school authorities, when rumblings about the inappropriateness of a curriculum are heard, is to rearrange the content to silence discontent. Often what results is what Harnack (quoted by Abrahamson) calls 'a rearrangement of the deck chairs on the Titanic'.[3]

As Dressel points out, a mere reorganisation of subject matter does not necessarily restore unity to an otherwise disjointed and disintegrated curriculum.[1]

The total educational experience should add up to something which the learner perceives as unity. That perception is effected for the individual learner by emphasising the relationships not only among different subjects but also between preceding and present learning in a given subject. Integration involves harmonising existing learning with new learning.

The term 'synchronisation' is used here to indicate the simultaneous teaching of closely related content. Harden, in his integration ladder summarised later in this chapter, refers to this as 'temporal coordination'.[4] This does not necessarily imply that the learner is exposed to all related content in the same learning experience. Practical considerations preclude such a strategy even with the best team-teaching efforts. In the medical curriculum, where so many closely related content areas interdigitate, it would be well-nigh impossible to achieve that degree of synchronisation. However, synchronising the teaching of related content within the same curriculum unit or block is a real possibility. This practice has given rise to the notion of 'block teaching' in medical education. Many attempts at integration merely result in synchronised block teaching. The essential ingredient, correlation, is often lacking, resulting in an experience that could hardly be said to be integrated. If synchronised teaching is to be effective as an integrating strategy it is imperative that the teachers who participate in such endeavours communicate with one another in the planning stages of the exercise and ensure that they are not only aware of one another's contributions but also take adequate steps to reinforce one another's individual efforts by highlighting the relationships among them. While well-planned team teaching may increase the chances of this occurring, it is not a *sine qua non* of integration.

A particular difficulty faced by teachers who attempt synchronised teaching is inequality among different disciplines of volume of content in a given course unit. For example, if the unit of integration is the organ system, anatomy may have more content in the musculo-skeletal system than either physiology or pathology, and physiology and anatomy more than pathology in the nervous system. Curricula that have commenced with laudable intentions of integration have regressed to subject-centred ones as teachers become frustrated by attempts to fit uneven content into a rigid timetable. The problem has arisen because of two factors: the reluctance of departments to relinquish ownership of pieces of the curriculum and an insistence on consistency in weekly scheduled time for each discipline in the programme. Significant integration of any form is unlikely to succeed unless teachers learn to work together, irrespective of departmental affiliations, and accept ownership of curricular units at multi-departmental rather than uni-departmental levels. This would involve a certain amount of 'give and take' in regard to curricular time, as well as flexibility in timetabling from one week to another.

Closely related to synchrony in teaching is contiguity, where similar material presented side by side enhances learning by helping the learner to see the similarities. Continuity in teaching, on the other hand, refers to the sequence in which material is presented. A correct sequence involves not only the logical arrangement of content within a single discipline but also the opportunity to relate material in one discipline to corresponding parts of another. Often teachers feel obliged to cover the content within a given area, with little concern for establishing the relationships with content presented by others. The teacher who is concerned with facilitating integration would pay particular attention to the transition from one topic to another, be it within his own field or related fields.

The medical curriculum is traditionally sequenced from normal to abnormal structure and function followed by clinical application. While it is essential to learn concepts pertaining to a relationship before the latter is learnt, postponement of that relationship to a later phase may result in forgetting the related concepts. As medical teachers have increasingly realised the need to demonstrate application of the theoretical concepts as soon as possible after they are learnt, the curricular sequence has gradually changed to enable the patient to be introduced to the student fairly early in the curriculum. Curriculum planners in many medical schools have heeded the criticisms levelled at the traditional practice of confining students to the study of cadavers from their first year in medical school. Instead, opportunities are increasingly being provided for the application of the basic sciences on the living, both normal and abnormal. In addition the basic sciences are reinforced at an applied level by clinical teachers in the latter phases of the curriculum, providing continuity of learning among the sequential phases of the curriculum. The integration of learning of basic and clinical sciences has been greatly enhanced by these practices.

The degree of integrating behaviour that the learner is called upon to demonstrate depends on two factors: the extent to which the teacher does the integrating activity and the extent to which the learner attempts to relate formal learning to everyday life. In regard to the former, Krathwohl has identified three levels of integration.[5]

1 The learner assimilates a completely developed scheme or pattern derived by the teacher.
2 The learner discovers the pattern selected by the teacher with some help from the latter.
3 The learner identifies a pattern by himself.

Although Krathwohl identifies these three levels, they are in fact points on the 'integrated-integrating' continuum, which was discussed in Chapter 1. A learning experience that enhances integration could fall anywhere along this continuum depending on the degree of freedom available to the learner to undertake his own integrations. Most of the strategies already referred to, such as continuity, sequencing, synchronisation and team teaching are predominantly teacher-directed. While they undoubtedly enhance integrated learning they do not guarantee that the learner develops skills in integrating what he learns, as they focus on the process of teaching rather than on what occurs in the mind of the learner. The learner who makes his own correlations, however, moves on the continuum towards integrating behaviour.

All the methods of integration already outlined depend on the manner in which curricular content is organised or presented to the learner. The second factor on which the level of integrated learning depends derives from the relationship between the internal and external environments of the learner, the extent to which the learner's 'heart . . . head and . . . hand work together'. On this basis, Megroth and Washburne identify three levels of integrated learning.[6]

1 The learner perceives relationships among elements outside him. For example, he sees a relationship between the method of science and clinical diagnosis. He constantly perseveres to integrate curricular learning to the external environment.

2 The learner attempts to perceive relationships in the internal environment, relating his knowledge to his attitudes and feelings. When he recognises contradictions the integrating learner will deal with them rather than explain them away through rationalisation. The learner who is unable to achieve significant integration at this level will 'clutch at straws' in the external environment to explain his perception of the internal environment. For example, a medical student who, when faced with a non-communicative patient from whom he is unable to extract a history, may blame the patient's communication skills if his integrative capacity at this level is low. Another student who is able to achieve significant integration at this level will reconcile his lack of skills in communication with this particular patient with his feelings for the patient's helplessness, and will take the appropriate steps to give of his utmost to the patient's cause.

3 At the third level, the learner attempts to synthesise all his experiences, both internal and external to himself, integrating his intellectual activity with other aspects of his life. Facts are not learnt just for their own sake, but are related to present or future life. At this level, disharmony between intellectual activity and the external environment could result in confusion to the learner who is unable to achieve significant integration. This is the level of integration that is, perhaps, most important in medical school, as this is where relationships between present learning and future professional practice need to be emphasised.

These three levels can be demonstrated further with an example relevant to learning in medical school. The medical student learns, in several disciplines in the curriculum, about the need for avoidance of contamination with organisms to prevent cross-infection. At the first level, the integrating learner will be able to perceive the relationships in his learning of theory and practice – for instance, in microbiology, pathology and surgery. At the second level the integrating learner is able to harmonise that learning with his views about cleanliness, rather than explain away his dirty fingernails or ungainly hair. At the third level he is able to integrate his inner feelings and learning with the practices he sees in his environment and envisages his role in harmonising the internal and external environment in his present or future practice.

On the other hand, the learner who is less integrative at the first level may not see the relationships among the facts he learns in the different subjects; at the second level, he rationalises dirty fingernails in spite of his awareness of the risk of contamination they carry; and at the third level, he ignores, condones or sometimes even contributes to practices that are likely to lead to cross-infection, rather than taking corrective action. As Megroth and Washburne succinctly state, '[t]he teaching problem is to assist students to see the connections between living and learning'.[6]

The non-integrating learner places learning and life in separate compartments. When the learning task is done he removes the 'garb of learning' and dons the 'garb of living'. At times, for the medical student, this is part of an escape phenomenon. He dares not let his feelings for the cadaver he has just dissected, or for the terminally ill patient he has just examined, affect his daily life. So he puts up a barrier between his learning and living. Because of his inability to come to terms with his own feelings, he suppresses them to go on living normally or at least put on a facade of normality. The integrating learner, at the third level of classification by Megroth and Washburne, however, learns to cope with his feelings for the cadaver or the dying patient, and attempts to draw lessons from these experiences and to apply them to both learning and living.

MODELS OF INTEGRATION

A curriculum model provides guidance on the manner in which a curriculum can be planned. It is a template on which the plan is based. The SPICES model is a set of characteristics or themes of a curriculum, each of which is arranged in the form of a continuum, with one end being most desirable and the other being least desirable.[7] It informs curriculum planners on the desirable attributes of an undergraduate medical curriculum, even though it may not provide a method for curriculum planning. Curriculum planners are encouraged to move to the positive end of the continuum representing each attribute when planning the curriculum. One attribute has integration at the positive end and discipline-orientation at the negative end.

There is a feeling among some medical educators that integration can only occur if departmental barriers are abolished. In Chapter 1 it was shown that integration can occur even within a discipline-based medical school. The particular model on which integration in a medical curriculum is based depends to a large extent on the degree to which the department forms the organisational unit of the medical school and the degree of responsibility this unit has for parts of the curriculum. Some integrating models assume the existence of departments with power to plan and implement the curriculum; others assume the existence of departments but limit curricular function to interdepartmental bodies; still others do not assume the existence of departments except as administrative entities. The author is unaware of any medical school where departments have been totally abolished, even though Moritz (cited by Hartroft) stated as long ago as 1964:

> If we could look in a crystal ball and see departmental organization in medical schools ten years from now, I doubt we would find departments as they now exist. I can easily imagine that there will be a consolidation of present departments which will eliminate many of the administrative partitions that now separate teachers and investigators.[8]

Four and a half decades later, departments continue to exist, though only for administrative purposes in some medical schools.

Integrating practices can be classified into a hierarchy of planning, implementing and evaluating modes. This classification can be illustrated in the case of a school in which departments exist. In the planning mode, interdepartmental planning meetings will be held in which a given course is planned. The implementation of that plan and the evaluation of the students at the end of the course will then be left to the individual departments concerned. In the implementing mode, planning and implementation will be undertaken together by the departments concerned. Finally, in the evaluating mode, planning, implementation and evaluation are undertaken as interdepartmental ventures. As will be discussed in Chapter 6, it is obvious that the most effective of these hierarchical levels is the last, as assessment largely determines the manner in which students learn.

Mayhew identified four types of integrative concepts.[9]

1 'Additive', where courses are added 'one on top of each other'. It has been argued above that such addition, by itself, does not necessarily result in integration.
2 'Sampling', where each integrated course mirrors a greater whole.
3 'Relational', where autonomy of the parts of the course is preserved but there is a 'pluralistic wholeness' about the total course offering.
4 'Holistic', where the whole is greater than the sum of the parts (departments), and the function of each part is circumscribed by both the other parts and the whole.

These types contribute to different degrees of integration, and offer four conceptual models for the practical implementation of a curriculum. However, it must be realised that none of them results in integration unless planning is undertaken as a joint venture by those responsible for the several parts.

Organ coined the terms 'theoretical integration' (such as between different branches of knowledge) and 'practical integration' (between knowledge and action), and identified four models of theoretical integration.[10]

1 'Historical', where events are put together in chronological sequence. In the medical curriculum a typical example is embryology, which requires the student to learn events pertaining to the development of the embryo, or its parts, in chronological sequence.

2 'Encyclopaedic', where the wholeness of the subject matter is the prime concern, in order to enable the student to understand concepts. This type of integration is of increasing concern to basic scientists, who see the erosion of this wholeness within their particular science with the rise of innovative methods such as problem-based learning. It must be realised that each science has achieved encyclopaedic integration within it, the wholeness of which is what the basic scientist attempts to achieve.

3 'Methodological', which focuses on the manner in which knowledge is gained, such as through experience or through the process of solving problems.

4 'Conceptual', in which the concept becomes the organising principle.

Organ goes on to warn us that theoretical forms of integration are inadvisable in elementary education, where significant integrations are personal in nature, and theoretical forms are more likely to be the teacher's integration foisted on the learner. He suggests that, by the time the learner reaches his third decade of life, he would have formed theoretical integration of his own, often neither evident to the teacher nor tested, and the former is in a better position to convert such theoretical integration into a practical one. The issue as to whether integration at this stage should be left to the learner, rather than be foisted on him by the teacher, will be dealt with in Chapter 5, where the advantages and disadvantages of this practice will be examined more closely.

Learning experiences that place students in situations where they are called upon to apply their theoretical concepts to practice will encourage practical integration. The term *practice* as used here is not synonymous with psychomotor skill, but applies to any activity that the student engages in, either in professional life or in preparation for that. Since a physician is always engaged in solving problems, learning opportunities that call upon the medical student to apply his knowledge to the solution of problems, which he is likely to encounter in professional life, encourage practical integrated learning.

Harden depicted the continuum of integration in the form of a ladder, with several intermediate steps between the extremes of the continuum: integration – discipline orientation.[4] This ladder provides a useful guide to curriculum

Transdisciplinary – "real world" situations

Interdisciplinary – loss of discipline perspective

Multidisciplinary – many subjects together

Complementary – focus on themes, topics

Correlation – only areas of common interest

Sharing – joint teaching

Temporal Coordination – synchronization

Nesting – infusion with elements of other subjects

Harmonization – connection, consultation, subject-based

Awareness – subject-based but aware of others' contributions

Isolation – fragmentation, subject-based

FIGURE 3.1 The integration ladder[4]

planners to determine the extent of integration they can expect to achieve given the specific circumstances they are faced with.

Of the 11 steps in the ladder, the lowest four rungs are strictly confined to disciplines, the next six rungs cut across disciplines and the last is the highest level of integration, where the student takes responsibility for integrated learning. The steps are summarised as the following 11 points.

1 *Isolation* or **fragmentation**, which is the traditional subject centred curriculum, where teachers in a given subject pay little attention to what goes on in other subjects.

2 In the next stage, *awareness*, the teacher in a given subject may become aware of what is taught in other related subjects, but without consulting teachers of the latter.

3 In the stage of *harmonisation*, teachers from different disciplines consult one another and, as a result of this, a teacher in a given subject may make connections to related parts of other subjects.

4 In *nesting*, the teacher in a given subject may deliberately include content from other subjects to enrich her own.

5 *Temporal coordination* refers to the practice of timing concurrently related courses in consultation with the teachers of those courses, to facilitate integrated learning by the students. This practice has been called 'synchronisation' by the author (*see*, p. 25).

6 *Sharing* or joint teaching (referred to earlier as team teaching) is when two or more departments jointly plan and implement a teaching unit.

7 In *correlation*, while the emphasis may still remain on the disciplines, additional courses that bring together areas of common interest to many disciplines are included.

8 At the level of *complementary* integration there is a mix of subject-based and integrated courses, with the focus of the latter on themes or topics.

9 *Multidisciplinary* integration occurs when subject areas are brought together in a course that centres on such themes as health problems, body organ systems, the life cycle or on special topics such as medical ethics.

10 *Interdisciplinary* education is similar except that no reference is made at all to the individual disciplines, which remain largely unidentifiable.

11 Finally, *transdisciplinary* integration transcends disciplines in a way that the focus is on a field of knowledge in the real world, which the student integrates in his own mind, with the help of a framework provided by the teacher.

While the last level is what we hope to achieve in all forms of integration, as discussed in Chapter 1, it becomes obvious that as teachers ascend the ladder they are increasingly likely to attain the goal of students undertaking integration for themselves in their own minds.

A useful classification of integrated learning experiences, which lends itself to models for the medical curriculum, is that of horizontal and vertical integration. As these terms have sometimes been used interchangeably, it is important at the outset to define them.

Benor identifies six parameters within the methods available for integration:[11]

1 the scope of integration (i.e. the number of disciplines involved and the extent of links among them)

2 the timing of integration within the curriculum

3 the environment in which learning takes place

4 the domains of learning involved (i.e. knowledge, skills and attitudes)

5 the students' role in the integrating process

6 the direction of interdisciplinary integration.

The last parameter refers to the notions of horizontal and vertical integration.

In the context of the undergraduate medical curriculum, horizontal integration refers to linking disciplines that, in a conventional curriculum, are taught at a given stage. Thus linking the basic medical science subjects of anatomy, physiology and biochemistry would be an example of horizontal integration. Vertical integration, on the other hand, refers to the linking of subjects that are conventionally taught at different stages. Thus linking anatomy with pathology and surgery would be an example of vertical integration. This classification is illustrated in Figure 3.2.

The horizontal model enables the learner to perceive the inter-relationships among concepts, principles and factual information that he is learning at the time, so that he understands phenomena in a holistic manner. For example, he learns the gross appearance of the kidney, understands how the kidney was formed and came to be where it is situated, recognises the intricate structure of

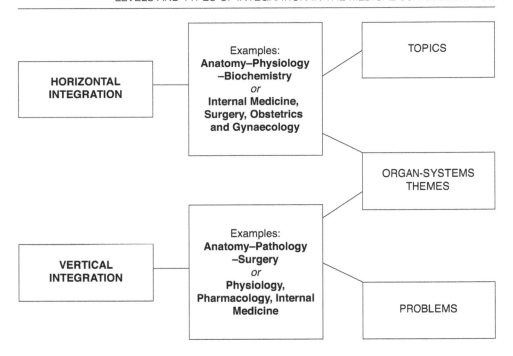

FIGURE 3.2 Horizontal and vertical integration

its different parts at microscopic and submicroscopic levels and relates that to the manner in which it functions and preserves the chemical composition and physical properties of the body fluids. He has obtained a holistic picture of the normal kidney. In vertical integration, he is encouraged to relate that picture of normality to deviations from the normal, and to perceive the changes that occur in the kidney by way of both structural alteration and dysfunction, the effects of such dysfunction on the composition of body fluids and how external agents can correct such dysfunction. Further vertical integration would result in an appreciation of the effects of such dysfunction on the patient by way of the signs and symptoms it produces, the differentiation of that dysfunction from conditions that produce similar signs and symptoms and suggesting the manner in which the patient with such dysfunction can be managed.

It can thus be seen that vertical integration enables the learner to apply directly and immediately the concepts, principles and factual information he has gained. This follows two well-known educational principles:

1 perception of relevance motivates and enhances learning
2 immediate application enhances long-term memory.

However, complete vertical integration, as in the previous example relating to the kidney, is rarely achieved in the medical curriculum, due to logistic difficulties arising from clinical care and patient availability, which will be pointed out in the next chapter.

The outlined discussion also indicates that both horizontal and vertical integration can be achieved to different degrees in the medical curriculum. This reflects the first of Benor's parameters of integration – namely, the extent of integration,[11] one aspect of which was discussed at the beginning of this chapter. This parameter will be examined more closely in relation to horizontal and vertical integration.

Benor contends that the extent of integration depends on both the number of subjects linked and the number of links between pairs of subjects. In horizontal integration, for example, structure may be linked with function but chemical composition may be excluded or included. In vertical integration, structure and function may be linked with dysfunction but the effects of dysfunction on the patient and the management of the patient may be excluded or included. On the other hand, only a few pairs of subjects may be linked within a curriculum, but they are so closely attached, through many relationships, that the degree of integration is increased. It is obvious that, if integrated learning is a desired outcome, the greater the number of subjects linked, and the greater the number of links among them, the more likely it is that the outcome will be achieved.

The distinction between competency-based and integrated curricula,[12] justified on the grounds that a competency-based curriculum is organised around functions that the professional undertakes in practice, and on the assumption that students learn to master prescribed objectives derived from these functions, is a mistaken one (*see* Chapter 1). The main characteristic of competency-based curricula is the manner in which the objectives of the curriculum are derived. Once this is achieved learning can be directed to those competencies identified, but such learning can take place in an integrated manner. Thus a competency-based curriculum can be integrated as well. For example, one integrated curriculum linked final-year theory objectives to practice objectives derived from job descriptions. Objectives for each year of the curriculum were derived from the succeeding year. Within each year integration was achieved through links among the subjects. In another, competency-based objectives were the main thrust of an integrated curriculum, which included essential competencies in its core, as well as problem-solving skills.[13] While any model should ideally aim to increase the links among its component parts, if the purpose of the curriculum is to prepare the student for future professional life, the curriculum should undoubtedly be directed towards those competencies that the professional is called upon to display in that life.

ORGANISING THEMES AND INTEGRATING THREADS

Any form of arrangement or grouping of content in a curriculum must be based on an organising theme that gives meaning to the structure of the curriculum. Elements of the curriculum that are significant for a given field within it, as well as to the entire curriculum, must be identified as the basis for organising the curriculum.

In the traditional medical school the organising theme for the entire curriculum is the disciplines or subjects. These are logical, meaningful entities into which the expanding knowledge has been compartmentalised. The organising theme within each subject differs from one subject to another. Thus content in gross anatomy is divided according to body regions, as this is seen as a logical way in which the student could dissect and learn about the anatomical relationships within the body. On the other hand, the content in organogenesis (development of the organs) is arranged according to organ systems, as that permits a logical and practical exposition of the manner in which each system was formed, even though development of the systems occurs approximately concurrently. Such an arrangement is quite different from that adopted for embryogenesis (early development of the embryo before the organ systems are laid down), which is best learnt in a chronological sequence commencing from the fertilised ovum. The same chronological sequence is followed within each organ system. Embryology is an unfolding story, starting with conception and ending with the fully formed foetus. The story must be told from beginning to end, if it is to have meaning. But for ease of understanding, the story pertaining to each organ system is told separately. The integrating learner will be able to see the relationships among the separate stories, which may overlap chronologically.

While traditional curricula are subject-centred, an analysis of the objectives of such a curriculum usually reveals certain strands within it. One such set of strands is basic, clinical, community and behavioural sciences (*see* Case Study 3 in Chapter 9). The thickness of each strand may vary in the different parts of the curriculum. The stronger they are in each the greater the opportunities for integration among them.

In determining organising themes for the medical curriculum it must be realised that teacher and student perspectives about what they teach and learn, respectively, may differ. Teachers have specialised along a certain line, and see their speciality as a meaningful whole. They see an intrinsic organisation within the subject that the students may not see. Students come with a variety of life experiences that make sense to them, whereas the organisation of the subject itself does not. The conventional curriculum is organised along lines that are meaningful to teachers, and into which students are weaned only after they are exposed to the curriculum. Premature exposure of students to this intrinsic organisation may condition them to accept it, precluding them from developing their own organisational frameworks within the subject.[14] Organising themes that are more meaningful to students as they commence the curriculum enhance integrated learning. For example, a theme such as 'man and his environment' would be meaningful to the student even as he commences the curriculum, because he has experience of man's environment.

Organising themes for curricula that purport to be integrated have been varied. The first contemporary medical school to seriously introduce a curriculum that was more integrated than the conventional one was Western Reserve, where the 'organ system' was used as the theme for integration. Thus content within the curriculum was grouped, not according to the disciplines, but according to organ systems, within each of which subject content was regrouped from the conventional curriculum. Organ systems, however, are not inclusive enough to cover all aspects of a medical curriculum, as many areas of importance do not fall neatly within any of the systems. Thus curricula that use organ systems as the organising theme have a supplementary theme, which is covered by the general rubric 'topics'.

Another organising theme is a chronological one, which relates to temporal developments. This is of particular use in learning about the development of the human being, where the sequential progression from the cell to the embryo, foetus, child, adolescent, adult and the aged is evident to both teachers and students. The same principle can be applied in the clinical field to the progression from prevention, acquisition, complications, cure and rehabilitation in relation to a given disease. Another chronological theme is the natural history of a disease – that is, its pathogenesis and resolution. Chronological themes, while appropriate for some parts of a medical curriculum, are also not adequately inclusive, and must be combined with other themes.

An organising theme used by an increasing number of schools is the health problem. In those curricula that adopt problem-based learning, health problems form the nuclei around which learning takes place. While they are organising themes for curricular content, the problems themselves must be arranged and sequenced in some logical, meaningful manner. Most schools that espouse this type of curriculum use as the main organising theme the body organ systems, within each of which problems form the integrative threads. Integrative threads are links connecting separately taught subjects. Bloom suggested that effective integrative threads should:

➤ be useful across a variety of problems or questions
➤ lend themselves to alteration, improvement and extension in the future
➤ relate past experience to present
➤ be comprehensive to extend across the content of the subject
➤ be meaningful and useful to the student
➤ permit comparison and contrast of seemingly unrelated experiences.[15]

Problems can serve another important integrating function, as pointed out in Chapter 1. In a curriculum that is phased according to the developmental level of the student, a previously used problem can be reintroduced at an increasingly complex level as the student develops. This is known as the spiralling problem, and it helps to link old learning to new, one of the criteria laid down by Bloom.

A third way in which a problem enhances integration is through its potential to link content covered by different themes. For example, some problems transcend many organ systems into which the curriculum is divided, and dealing with them helps the student to establish links among these systems. In fact, some curricula have a unit named 'multi-systems unit' that deliberately introduces problems, such as diabetes mellitus, that have this potential across organ systems.

Problem-based curricula perhaps reach the acme of integration, if the problems that integrate are real-life problems that the student is likely to encounter in future professional life.

Tyler considered the 'warp' and the 'woof' of the curriculum fabric.[16] Concepts (such as interdependence among cells, systems or individuals), skills (such as problem solving) and values (such as primary healthcare) form the vertical warp of the fabric. The elements used at a horizontal level across the curricular strands, for example organ systems, form its woof. The tighter the links and knots in the fabric the stronger is the integrative support given by the fabric of the curriculum to sustain the student in its meshes.

KEY POINTS

- All curricula have some inherent degree of integration as 'part' and 'whole' are relative terms.
- Correlating or linking elements is the key to effective integration.
- Synchronisation and team teaching aid integration but do not guarantee it without the linking of subjects.
- The more the teacher integrates for the learner, the less the learner learns to integrate for himself.
- The highest integration is when the learner harmonises learning with living.
- Integrating learning experiences place students in situations where they apply theoretical concepts learnt in practice.
- In horizontal integration linking occurs among subjects learnt at the same level; in vertical integration, at different levels.

REFERENCES

1 Dressel PL. The meaning and significance of integration. In: Henry NB, editor. *The Integration of Educational Experiences*, 57th Yearbook of the National Society for the Study of Education, Part III. Chicago, IL: University of Chicago Press; 1958, Chapter XII, pp. 251–63.

2 Abrahamson S. Myths and shibboleths in medical education. *Teach Learn Med.* 1989; **1**: 4–9.

3 Abrahamson S. Changing curriculum in the medical school. *J Med Educ.* 1977; **52**: 778–9.

4 Harden RM. The integration ladder: a tool for curriculum planning and evaluation. *Med Educ.* 2000; **34**: 551–7.

5 Krathwohl DR. The psychological bases for integration. In: Henry NB, editor. *The Integration of Educational Experiences*, op. cit., Chapter III, pp. 43–65.

6 Megroth EJ, Washburne VZ. Integration in education. *J Educ Res.* 1949; **43**: 81–92.

7 Harden RM, Sowden S, Dunn WR. Educational strategies in curriculum development: the SPICES model. *Med Educ.* 1984; **18**: 284–97.

8 Hartroft WS. Physiology in pathology. *Lab Invest.* 1964; **13**: 602–9.

9 Mayhew LB. Illustrative courses and programs in colleges and universities. In: Henry NB, editor. *The Integration of Educational Experiences*, op. cit., Chapter XI, pp. 218–48.

10 Organ TW. Integration in higher education. *J Higher Educ.* 1955; **26**: 180–6.

11 Benor DE. Interdisciplinary integration in medical education: theory and method. *Med Educ.* 1982; **16**: 355–61.

12 McGaghie WC, Miller GE, Sajid AW, *et al.* Competency-based curriculum development in medical education: an introduction. *Public Health Pap.* 1978; **68**: 11–91.

13 Katz J, Fulop T. Personnel for health care: case studies of educational programmes. *Public Health Pap.* 1978; **70**: 1–260.

14 Capehart BE. Illustrative courses and programs in selected secondary schools. In: Henry NB, editor. *The Integration of Educational Experiences*, op. cit., Chapter X, pp. 194–217.

15 Bloom BS. Ideas, problems and methods of inquiry. In: Henry NB, editor. *The Integration of Educational Experiences*, op. cit., Chapter V, pp. 84–104.

16 Tyler RW. Curriculum organization, In: Henry NB, editor. *The Integration of Educational Experiences*, op. cit., Chapter VI, pp. 105–25.

CHAPTER 4

Integrative practices in the medical curriculum

According to Dressel, integrative practices generally fall into three categories:

1 those that develop interrelationships among existing courses
2 those that reorganise content into more general courses
3 those that arrange content around vital problems relevant to student or society.[1]

Many attempts at integration in the medical curriculum have included combinations of these three basic types.

This chapter summarises experiences reported in the literature, as well as those that the author has experienced himself, through direct involvement, through indirect involvement as a consultant or through observation during visits. The experiences will be divided into six categories:

1 component-focused integration, where the focus of integration is a particular component of the curriculum
2 horizontal integration involving a significant part of the curriculum
3 vertical integration, also involving a significant part of the curriculum
4 problem-centred integration, which belongs to Dressel's third category
5 community-based integration, where the locus of integration is the community
6 multiprofessional integration, where learning takes place with students from other health professions
7 integration of the art and science of medicine.

It is recognised that there is much overlap among these categories. However, there are also such significant differences, which impact heavily on the manner in which the business of the curriculum is carried out, that separate consideration is desirable.

Irrespective of the type of integration used, it is of paramount importance that integration in the student's learning, rather than in the teacher's teaching, be uppermost in the minds of both planners and implementers. The student should be motivated to display integrative behaviours and seek her own integrative links, rather than merely be exposed to the links displayed by the teacher. Motivation is heightened if the student can see wider application of the links to both daily life and future learning. The less structured the curriculum the greater is the integrative activity on the part of the student.[2] The secret is to 'whet, not satiate, the [student's] integrative appetite'.[1]

COMPONENT-FOCUSED INTEGRATION

In Chapter 1 the curriculum was described as a system consisting of interrelated components. It was also stated there that the curriculum is both a plan and a process. Dressel combined these thoughts in identifying the basis for promoting integration when he stated that there were four elements within a curriculum that could be so used: agreement on objectives, selection of a set of learning experiences, the organisation of those experiences and the process of evaluation.[1] While each of these elements is in itself complex, such categorisation is a logical basis on which to address the concept and practice of component-focused integration.

Integration is greatly hampered by a lack of agreement on the objectives of the curriculum among the various players. First, agreement between the planners and the implementers is essential if the curriculum on paper is to match that in practice. Second, agreement among the implementers themselves is critical if an integrated experience is to be given to the students. Third, however integrated the experience may be, if the students are either not clear about or do not agree with the objectives formulated by teachers, integrated learning will be endangered.

The objectives of a curriculum vary in both level and specificity. At one end of the spectrum are the overall goals and philosophy of the curriculum, often referred to as institutional goals. Institutional goals are usually quite explicitly stated and available in curricular documents published and advertised by the school. Experience has shown, however, that teachers are often either unaware of their institutional goals or, if they are aware, do not necessarily agree with them. Often they paint the curriculum in favourable colours, but the facade is easily penetrated when one visits the school for the first time and observes the real curriculum in practice, or when one questions the faculty members closely about what their real goals are. A typical example is related to the common goal of most medical schools that profess to train a 'basic doctor who is able to specialise along any branch of medicine after graduation from medical school'. Faculty members may have accepted that goal in formal meetings, but many teachers have not internalised it and continue to train medical students as though they were training clones of their own speciality. This practice is particularly common among basic science teachers. If there is an overt or covert lack of agreement, or unawareness, of the philosophy of the school, integration must necessarily be hampered. Implicit goals are more powerful than explicit goals. If a discrepancy exists between explicit and implicit goals, the organisation of learning experiences is not consistent and the experiences are not effectively integrative. On the other hand, if they coincide, they could result in very potent integration.[3]

At the next level are departmental objectives, in schools where the department has jurisdiction over a segment of the curriculum; or phase, unit or system objectives, in schools where the curriculum is interdepartmental. In the former, as long as departments agree with one another and work towards a common goal, integration is likely to succeed; if they do not, integration in the students' minds will be inversely proportional to the extent to which departments jockey for power within the curriculum. And power in the curriculum is usually equated with such factors as curriculum time, examination space, budgetary allocation and perceived importance. When students sacrifice one discipline for the sake of another, integration is jeopardised. In the second type of school, where the curriculum is interdepartmental, if dissonance exists in the general objectives of its various segments by way of undue relative emphases or content detail, student learning is determined by their perception of importance, not for practice, but for success at examinations. Integration is again in jeopardy.

At the third and most specific level are the objectives within each subject or unit. When such objectives are confined to single subjects or content areas, and not to the links among them, integration is de-emphasised, and student learning is piecemeal. While such objectives are inevitable in any curriculum, it is as important to include those that link the different subject and content areas, if integration is to be enhanced. As Pace points out, 'the potency of an objective in organising [student] behavior . . . [is] not identical with the potency of the objective in producing integrating behavior'.[3] Simple, immediate and very specific or detailed objectives have much less potential to produce integrative learning than those that are complex and long-term. He suggests three types of objectives that promote integrative learning behaviour:

1 those that require the student to link subject areas or knowledge to real-life experiences and problems
2 those that require the student to relate specific facts to broad principles and generalisations
3 those that involve the intellect and feelings, beliefs and values.

He points out the integrative nature of objectives which promote critical thinking as they require the learner to call upon knowledge from related disciplines or courses. Creativity goes even a step further in that it calls upon the individual to relate seemingly unrelated items to come up with something new. Koestler used the term 'bisociation' for this type of creative activity.[4]

Dressel's second curriculum element that can be used to promote integration is the selection of learning experiences.[1] Many are the descriptions in the literature of attempts to increase integration in the undergraduate medical curriculum by focusing on the selection of methods. It should be stated at the outset that many attempts to achieve integration have failed to do so simply because adequate attention has not been given to the first requirement – namely, agreement on objectives. One classic example of this futile emphasis on method is the most inappropriately named 'block lecture', which consists of a series of mini-lectures given by three or four teachers from different disciplines on a given topic, without ever having discussed the nature of their inputs with each other, and often without even arriving at consensus on the objectives of their inputs. As a result, students are exposed to a succession of disjointed inputs, which do little to enhance their integrative behaviour. Even some problem-based schools pursue this practice under the guise of 'fixed resource sessions' or 'fixed learning modules', a euphemism for a series of mini-lectures to 'cover' the subject as fast as possible. Guilbert labelled this latter practice 'coveritis',[5] a disease perhaps missed out by Abrahamson in his witty paper entitled 'Diseases of the Curriculum'.[6]

The organisation of integrative learning experiences requires much more thought and planning than it is customarily accorded. Integration does not take place because of any particular method or curricular organisation, unless that method or organisation encourages the student to undertake integrative activity, be it intellectual or experiential.

Benor identifies case presentations, clinical application, simulations and the solving of diagnostic and management problems as methods used to enhance integration.[2] The ubiquitous clinico-pathological conference has the potential to be a powerful integrative method, if only it does not degenerate into a battle of wits between specialists, with each trying to outdo the other, forgetting the student in the process.[7] Similar to the great books seminars practised by the masters of yore in teaching literature,[3] medical school teachers have developed interdisciplinary workbooks that not only safeguard the integrated character of the programme but also require the student to practise integration through exercises and quizzes testing links among the subjects.

In organising learning experiences, integration is enhanced through the use of appropriate learning venues. The visitor to the McMaster University's School of Medicine in Hamilton, Ontario, would be perplexed at the way in which the clinical wards, laboratories and classrooms blend with one another. The use of the multidisciplinary laboratory is another attempt to use the locus of learning to enhance integration.[8] Here the preclinical student has an assigned space within a laboratory used by all the disciplines, and the laboratory is brought to the student instead of the student going to each of them. Katz and Fulop point out several examples of the use of multidisciplinary laboratories and their advantages for preclinical learning.[9] The anatomy museum, a bastion of traditional departments of this subject, can be reorganised in a way that promotes integration both within and between problems in a problem-based curriculum.[10] As will be discussed in the section on community-based integration later in this chapter, the locus of learning plays a crucial part in integration. The sole dependence on any one method or medium ultimately demands consideration of other methods and media if integration is to improve.[11]

The last element identified by Dressel as a basis for promoting integration is assessment.[1] This important component deserves separate consideration, and will be addressed in Chapter 6. It will be shown there that, whatever strategy the teacher may use to integrate teaching, if integrated learning is to take place the component of the curriculum with which students are most concerned should not be neglected. Attempts to integrate the curriculum in the face of 'disintegrated' examinations are bound to fail, as far as the students are concerned. Hence it is necessary to consider this component separately.

HORIZONTAL INTEGRATION

Horizontal integration can occur at both preclinical and clinical levels within the medical curriculum. The conventional preclinical curriculum is based on a 'code' established by each department, with definite boundaries that may or may not include the student's personal experience of the world.[12] A recent experience brought this home quite clearly to the author, while teaching anatomy. A demonstration using a cadaver specimen to a group of students on the anatomy of the female reproductive system was interrupted by the sudden gasp of a female student. On inquiring about the reason for this expression of surprise, the student revealed that she could not imagine how such a relatively large full-term baby could be accommodated in such a small uterus! In spite of the fact that the student would have seen numerous pregnant women whose abdomens increased in size as pregnancy advanced, she could not fathom that the uterus was increasing in size to accommodate the growing foetus. This was the starting point for this student's learning, if she was to integrate her personal life experience with the content she was about to learn. If she were merely exposed to the structure and relationships of the uterus, she would not have been able to integrate her experience with the new learning, and would not have been encouraged to make that link, except through subsequent reflection. The latter is the desirable practice of reflective learning, but it would undoubtedly be of benefit to all students to relate the size of the uterus to its function, through the judicious use of questions at the outset of learning the anatomy of the uterus. This is in fact horizontal integration. It is a means by which principles and facts from several related disciplines appropriate to the level at which the student is learning are selected, organised and linked to one another in a manner that fills in the gaps in the student's mind and creates a more complete picture.

Bloom suggests that, for effective integration to take place, students must have the opportunity to relate educational experiences that are taking place in close proximity to one another.[13] The conventional medical curriculum rarely heeds this advice, as often structure and function are dissociated. For example, preclinical students may learn the anatomy of the upper limb concurrently with the physiology of the heart. By the time they learn muscle function and the structure of the heart, respectively, they would have forgotten, or would pay scant attention to, their former learning, and are thus not encouraged to make the links between structure and function. Synchronisation, the term used to describe the practice of teaching related content from different disciplines concurrently, facilitates linking, but is not the sole requirement for integration. Synchronisation without linking results in little integration.

Integration must begin in the teachers who, while specialists in their own discipline, are familiar with the contributions of colleagues in related parts of the curriculum. As the number of parts increases, the relationships among them increase exponentially, and integration becomes correspondingly more difficult. Consequently, as specialisation within the curriculum increases and the curriculum splinters into multiple components the extent of horizontal integration is likely to decrease. One can only speculate why this should be so. As the specialist becomes increasingly specialised, one would expect mastery of the sub-speciality, drawing from all related disciplines. Hence the reluctance to expose students to the links among the disciplines in that narrow area is incomprehensible. If all specialists were to adopt this practice of linking relevant content, horizontal integration would increase. Such an increase would be at the expense of integration among the various sub-speciality content areas. This requires someone with a broader vision of the discipline than that of the narrow specialist. As Armstrong pointed out, reductionism is a way of making explanations easier, as anatomical structure is reduced to histology, physiological phenomena to biochemical events and human behaviour to neurophysiological concepts.[12] He argues that such reductionism implies a false simplicity to natural phenomena that are multifactorial.

As a matter of fact no one discipline can isolate itself from the others, as knowledge used in one is both dependent and influential on the other disciplines. This is evident in the case of both preclinical and clinical disciplines. How could structure be *understood* without relating it to function, and vice versa? The understanding of basic concepts involves the integration of learning related to the basic functions of the human body.

One of the earliest attempts in an Asian country at interdisciplinary horizontal integration on a significant part of the preclinical medical curriculum was undertaken by the author in 1974 in the Peradeniya Medical School of the University of Sri Lanka. Known as the Cell Biology Project, it integrated content pertaining to the normal cell and involved teachers from the departments of anatomy, biochemistry, physiology and microbiology. Benor, in 1982, described a coordinated second-year course at Beersheba in Israel that integrated cellular and molecular biology of mammalian and bacterial cells, with contributions from physiology, immunology and genetics.[2] However, as late as 2001, medical academics were still bemoaning the lack of teaching in cell biology and exhorting the integration of this subject with the clinical sciences.[14]

The premedical curriculum usually caters to a mixed group of students who have entered a school for the study of medicine but have different academic backgrounds. In order to get them to a fairly uniform level of prerequisite abilities for the study of preclinical medicine, they are exposed to courses in the physical, chemical and biological sciences. Many of the concepts they learn are boringly repetitious for some, while for others they are frustratingly difficult. The root cause of the problem is inappropriate selection of students for admission. Much of the content is repeated in one form or another during their preclinical years. Recognising the futility of this unwarranted repetition of subject matter, some medical schools, such as that in the University of New South Wales in Sydney, have integrated the relevant components of the premedical sciences into the preclinical phase, heightening motivation from the perception of relevance, and saving time and resources that are in high demand during the period of undergraduate medical education. Gellhorn and Scheuer also report such an integrated course in the City College of New York.[15] Hayter describes how Robertson, Professor of Physics at the Queen's University in Canada, was able to integrate the pure and applied sciences of physics and radiology in one course as far back as 1920. The course was successfully implemented until 1964, when physics was made a requirement for entry to medical school and medical radiology was made a clinical rotation.[16]

On the clinical side, what is considered to be content in a given discipline, such as typhoid in internal medicine, has repercussions on surgery (typhoid ulcer perforation), paediatrics (immunisation) and community medicine (spread). It would be far more meaningful for these clinical departments to collaborate in exposing the clinical student to this topic. Unfortunately, the separation of the clinical disciplines is as sharp as that among the preclinical disciplines. Often the clinical teacher forgets that the patient does not walk into the clinic of a primary care physician with a label on his back identifying him as a surgical or medical patient, but with an undifferentiated clinical problem.

One of the difficulties in horizontal integration during the clinical phase is a logistic one of getting a group of clinicians from different specialities together to undertake a joint teaching activity. While this is a real problem for busy clinicians, it was pointed out earlier that team teaching is not a *sine qua non* for integrated teaching. A surgeon teaching clinical students about dysphagia could, without much difficulty, expose them to its so-called 'medical' causes; so could an internist teaching about diabetes mellitus expose them to its so-called 'surgical' complications.

Kilminster *et al.* describe the use of specialised ward-based teachers, rather than consultants, to develop third-year medical students' clinical skills of history-taking and examination.[17] Several advantages of this strategy were perceived: overcoming the difficulties consultants have of providing sufficient supervision for medical students in the face of other competing demands for their time; overcoming the feeling of intimidation that beginning clinical students express when they are observed by consultants; and the potential for integrating ward-based clinical and clinical skills centre teaching, including standardisation of techniques. While the latter advantage certainly has merit, the practice may to some extent go against the concept of integration, as students may think it is not the consultant's role to undertake basic practical clinical skills.

A cluster of three clinical subjects has emerged in the present medical curriculum, which seems to lend itself well to integrated teaching – namely, community medicine, geriatric medicine and general practice. Stout and Irwin described a course at Queen's University in Belfast that has added a fourth subject, mental health, to this trio.[18] They were all subjects that shared a common theme of hospital and community care and of management of the patient within his environment. Furthermore these subjects usually fell within the ambit of a couple of departments, making horizontal integration easier. Topics within these subjects were each discussed in student groups over about half a day, led by a teacher who was a member of the academic staff, a consultant, a general practitioner or a member of the paramedical staff. In addition to this integrated course, each department had its own teaching programme. This is a practical strategy for schools that attempt to increase the degree of integration, but are reluctant to extend it across the entire curriculum.

Wallace *et al.* described how an integrated clinical teaching programme between general practice and hospital clinical teaching, known as Community-Based Medical Education in North Thames (CeMENT), was planned and implemented in five London medical schools with widely differing curricula.[19] The programme was perceived by both students and teachers as providing the former with a balanced view of the presentation and management of illness.

'Curricular arthritis' sets in when communications patterns are affected and faculty are unable or unwilling to plan with each other.[6] Horizontal integration is severely affected.

VERTICAL INTEGRATION

In 1958, Krathwohl postulated a general educational theory that posits that those concepts that are important to develop a given relationship should be taught just before the relationship is established.[20] Clinical teachers, well aware of this necessity, often encourage medical students to recall the concepts, facts and principles they learnt in the basic sciences before they relate those concepts to one another in the context of a given patient. The common experience of clinical teachers, as judged by their oft-expressed complaint, is that most students either do not know or do not remember the basic science concepts that they learnt in an earlier phase of the curriculum. For the student that part of the curriculum has been overcome, as a hurdler overcomes each hurdle, and attention is now focused on the next hurdle. Unfortunately, each 'hurdle' in the medical curriculum is not an independent entity, but is built on the gains from overcoming the previous hurdle. Inevitably, the clinical teacher 'revises' the basic sciences with the students before the clinical concepts are taught, because they are prerequisite to the clinical concepts. If one analyses this common sequence of events, one would find that what is repeated are the basic science concepts, whereas they were merely aids to the learning of the concepts on which the practice of medicine is dependent.

Vertical integration is one means of overcoming this disadvantage to some extent. It is a means of relating educational experiences customarily taking place at different times in the curriculum, through the exposition of the application of the basic sciences at the time they are learnt, as well as at the time the clinical sciences are taught. In the former instance, the clinical application is exposed to the student for the purpose of motivation and longer retention, while the prime objective is the learning of the basic sciences. In the latter instance, the basic sciences are recalled as a means of understanding the basis of clinical practice, while the prime objective is the learning of the methods of clinical practice. In both instances vertical integration is achieved.

In the previous section, the value of horizontal integration was shown to be the holistic nature of the educational experience. Vertical integration, on the other hand, while adding another dimension to this wholeness, relates the learning to the future professional life of the student, the life that she envisages and for which she sees herself as preparing. Thus both horizontal and vertical integration are important dimensions in determining the cumulative and integrative effect of educational experiences.[21] When vertical integration is not emphasised students fail to see the application and usefulness of knowledge.

Christie states that, for vertical integration, a common language is necessary, and that very often the clinician is not 'talking the same language' as the physiologist or biochemist.[22] Both basic scientist and clinician must learn this common language and be able to identify with each other if vertical integration is to be successful. This is one reason why extensive vertical integration across a conventional curriculum is difficult. It is achieved to some extent in problem-based curricula, as will be discussed in the next section. Some degree of vertical integration is possible within the conventional curriculum, and many are the reports of efforts to do so.

From this discussion it is obvious that vertical integration can and should take place in both phases of the medical curriculum. It is not an uncommon practice for surgeons, particularly orthopaedic surgeons, to contribute to courses in anatomy, and for internists who have specialised in a particular field to contribute to courses in physiology and pharmacology. This may seem to imply that anatomy is more relevant to surgery and physiology to internal medicine. Such an association is obviously not an exclusive one. The student who is taught physiology by an internist, or anatomy by a surgeon, will not fail to be impressed as to the relevance of what she is learning when she sees the type of professional she envisages herself to be teaching that particular discipline. In a survey carried out on 100 academic radiology departments in the United States, Basset and Squire found that in one-third of them radiologists teach anatomy to medical students, either in anatomy courses or in radiology courses, or in both.[23] The clinician is better than a basic scientist in impressing on the student how basic science knowledge is applied in clinical practice.

In curricula that adopt an organ-systems approach to horizontal integration, relevant patient care experience would undoubtedly go a long way in impressing upon the student the significance of what she is learning at the time. Clinical expediency and opportunity, however, usually dictate otherwise. It is usually not logistically feasible to arrange such experiences for all students in the hospital setting, as priority has to be given to clinical clerks. However, it is quite feasible to bring the patients to the students in the academic centre, for demonstrating relevant symptoms and signs, provided the patient is not too ill. If a clinical correlation session could be held even once a week for preclinical students, learning would be all the more effective. Reluctance of basic scientists to undertake such activities usually stems from their lack of confidence in their ability to deal with matters clinical, particularly if they have not had clinical training themselves.

A trend that made its presence felt in the second half of the last century was the early introduction of the student to the patient. In some schools, even before this era, such exposure was in the form of a 'preclinical clerkship'. Experiences with this had not been very satisfactory, usually because of the low priority given, and even the disdain meted out, to the 'half-baked' doctor by clinical practitioners and senior colleagues. As the preclinical clerkship was phased out of most medical curricula, another experience took its place in the form of introductory courses in the first year of the curriculum. A survey of such courses revealed a spectrum of aims from developing communication to physical examination skills.

The mere exposure of the preclinical student to clinical situations may help create motivation for the study of medicine,[24] but does little to enhance integration of learning unless deliberate attempts are made by the teacher to link their current learning to what they would experience in the future as clinical students. Furthermore, as pointed out in the commentary on this approach by Kachur,[25] students may become bored very soon if they are treated as 'flies on the wall' repeatedly, and even the motivating function may be compromised.

A novel programme was described by MacLeod *et al.* in the Wellington School of Medicine, where students in their first clinical year were exposed to dying patients and required to reflect on their beliefs, assumptions and previous life experiences.[26] While such experiences help the future physician cope with death and dying, integration is enhanced in that the students attempt to harmonise previous learning in the affective domain with new learning brought on by such structured experiences.

The reverse form of vertical integration, where basic scientists are invited to participate in teaching in the clinical setting, rarely occurs. Perhaps clinicians feel they could undertake such teaching themselves more effectively, and do not need basic scientists. Or the latter are reluctant to do so themselves, as pointed out. This is unfortunate as it deprives the latter from seeing the effects of their labour, when the student is called upon to apply his learning. The relatively little attention given to the basic sciences in the later years of the curriculum only helps to perpetuate and exaggerate the dichotomy between the clinical and basic sciences. An attempt to correct this was made in one medical school that adopts a problem-based curriculum, through a course on applied aspects of anatomy given to senior students in the clerkship phase by teachers from that department.[27]

Thus far only integration between basic and clinical sciences has been discussed. Benor described a course at Ben-Gurion University in which the scientific knowledge base is closely integrated with the clinical sciences, the behavioural sciences and public health, using the case-study method of teaching.[2] Problem-based learning, which has antecedents in the case-study method espoused by Harvard Law School, affords the same opportunity for integration of all four streams: basic sciences, clinical sciences, behavioural sciences and public health.

PROBLEM-BASED INTEGRATION

Curricula that are essentially centred on clinical and community problems became increasingly popular in medical education in the last quarter of the last century. The innovation started by the McMaster University's School of Medicine in Hamilton, Ontario, in 1971, based on previous experiences in fields other than medicine, was followed closely by the State University of Limburg in Maastricht, the Netherlands, and the University of Newcastle in Australia in the 1970s. For a period, however, there seemed to be reluctance by medical schools the world over to follow these pioneering efforts, perhaps due to a dearth of clear evidence of the superiority of this innovative approach over the more traditional one. Some schools experimented with parallel tracks in which both innovative and traditional methods were implemented simultaneously, apparently providing opportunities for comparison between the two. However, as the medical school in the State University of Michigan, East Lansing, realised early (personal communication, 1982), such comparison was fraught with danger, as many confounding variables existed, particularly when students and teachers were given the opportunity to participate in the track of their choice. Logically and educationally, however, the innovative approach appeared to be superior, and satisfaction surveys showed that, after an initial period of apprehension and reluctance, both students and teachers who participated in this new approach were in favour of it. It was a matter of time before the strategy was emulated by schools in many countries, exhorted by bodies governing medical education such as the General Medical Council in the United Kingdom and the Australian Medical Council. At the turn of the century there were supposed to be about 100 schools in the world that had espoused this approach in one way or another, and numbers have been growing since.

As pointed out earlier, this approach to learning offered the potential to reach the acme of horizontal and vertical integration, as clinical and community problems formed the triggers for learning the links among and between the basic, clinical and behavioural sciences and community medicine. While the approach ostensibly promoted integrated learning, did the amount of such learning actually increase in students who followed such curricula? This depended to a great extent on the manner in which the curriculum was implemented. In some schools problem-based tutorials only nominally provided a venue for problem solving by students, with tutors playing an unduly prominent role in tutorials, not much different from the lectures that they had replaced. The author became acutely aware of this when, as a consultant to a school with such a curriculum, he was requested by the school authorities to undertake an evaluation of the actual implementation of the curriculum. In an unobtrusive observation of one tutorial, the monologue of the tutor was embarrassingly obvious, and certainly did not provide an opportunity for students to integrate their learning through the problem.

In other schools, while the first of a set of tutorials devoted to a given problem commenced with problem solving, the tutorials that followed were largely didactic in nature, often with minimal reference to the original problem. In still others students very soon analysed the problem in a way that led to a separation of the basic and clinical science subjects, followed by learning each of these disciplines as distinct entities without linking them. All these practices diminish the degree of integrated learning that the problem is supposed to promote. Thus Heylings's findings, through a postal survey of 28 anatomy departments in the United Kingdom, that 'Gross Anatomy was fully integrated in the problem-based curricula',[28] can only be confirmed by observing the curricula being implemented, rather than through a review of curricular documents. Prince et al. showed that problem-based learning does not result in a lower level of anatomical knowledge than more traditional educational approaches.[29] The issue here is not whether the intended curriculum was problem-based or not but, rather, if the students were learning gross anatomy in an integrated manner through the problems or as a separate discipline after each problem was presented to them.

The integrating problem has the potential to integrate curricular units, which in many instances are the body organ systems. Thus a given problem may impact on many organ systems, calling upon the students to link prior learning with present learning. The concept of the spiral problem, where the same problem is presented at increasingly complex levels in successive units of the curriculum, encourages such integration while reinforcing previous learning through application to new learning.

A given problem is not confined to concepts belonging to a single discipline. In formulating objectives for a given problem, the problem constructor must attempt to include objectives from several disciplines and a wide range of subject matter, if it is to serve as an effective integrative thread.[13] For example, Benor refers to a tumour biology course in Beersheba in which case histories incorporate concepts related to cell biology, virology, immunology, genetics, physiology, pathology, physics, pharmacology, behavioural sciences and clinical skills.[2] In order to attempt to solve the problem the student is necessarily called upon to link these concepts, thereby integrating their learning both horizontally and vertically.

As repeatedly pointed out in previous chapters, true integration must take place in the minds of the learner. In spite of well-constructed problems, which have the potential to bring about integrating behaviour on the part of the student, if they are not allowed to exercise their minds in finding links between concepts, the ultimate goal of producing a creatively integrating learner will not be achieved.[20] Integrated learning can be thwarted by the manner in which the problem is constructed, by the biases of the facilitator or by the manner in which the tutorial is carried out. Dressel states that premature organisation of knowledge when solving the problem may stifle the need to integrate.[1] Such premature organisation may be at the behest of the facilitator or initiated by the student group in order to conform to a familiar way of dealing with the problem. The student is then engaged more in the memorisation of principles and theories rather than in integrating the learning that should occur from the problem.

The facilitator who does not allow sufficient room for students to explore their ideas, but attempts to force his point of view, and supplies information, however relevant it may be, stifles the attempts by the students to determine links among the concepts they learn. The skilled facilitator is one who encourages blurring of boundaries among disciplines, both horizontally and vertically, without establishing links among them himself.[30] Repeated memorisation of facilitator-presented integrations reduces the challenging potential of the problem and does little to motivate the student to learn. The thrill of discovery, a hallmark of problem-based learning and one of the most potent stimuli to learning, is to a large extent negated by the information-giving facilitator. In many situations the facilitator, who is aware of the correct answers to the questions raised by the students, should refrain from providing them, but allow the students to determine them by themselves.

Even worse is the facilitator who insists on a particular point of view. In 1996 Glasgow University introduced a problem-based integrated medical curriculum, in which medical ethics and law formed a vertical theme running through the five years of the curriculum.[31] One of the objectives of this theme was to ensure that students were aware of their ethical and legal obligations in clinical reasoning. A facilitator who forces his point of view when dealing with ethical dilemmas, without allowing the students to explore the pros and cons of each possible course of action, would do little to promote integrative behaviour when those students are faced with similar situations in real life. A truly integrating experience is one that promotes a degree of flexibility in the learner to become self-reliant in adjusting to new experiences.[1]

Readiness is an important prerequisite for integrated learning. As the degree of readiness brought about by prior learning varies among learners, the capacity to undertake integrated learning also varies. Krathwohl surmises that there is an optimum level of conceptualisation for persons with different levels of mental ability.[20] These educational concepts have an important bearing on the practicalities of problem-based learning as a means of promoting integrated learning. As with all educational experiences directed towards student groups, rather than individual learners, problems have to be so constructed as to facilitate learning by the average student. Problems that are too easy, based on simple objectives that the average student has largely achieved already, cease to be stimulating as the amount of conceptual linking that he is called upon to make is relatively small. On the other hand, if the problem is too difficult for him, directed to objectives beyond his ability and readiness, he may experience frustration as he is called upon to use concepts that do not exist in his mind. If problems are to serve as integrative threads they must be carefully selected and constructed in reference to the students involved.[13] The problem constructor must ensure that not only is the goal of integration attainable but that the students have confidence that they can attain that goal.[20] Furthermore, problems encountered in real life and in lifelike situations, which require the student to apply learning that cuts across narrow subjects, and that are perceived by the student to be important for him, are more likely to enhance integrated learning. This is in line with Schmidt's second element of information-processing theory underlying problem-based learning – namely, encoding – where the more closely the situation in which something is learnt resembles the situation in which it will be applied, the more likely is it that transfer of learning will occur.[32] While almost all clinical education occurs in the more contextually relevant process of patient care, the same is not true of basic science education, which is often divorced from patient care. Problem-based learning affords the student the opportunity to learn the basic sciences in a situation that is as close as possible to the situation where clinical learning occurs, without the practical difficulties associated with teaching the basic sciences in real patient contexts. Such practical difficulties are in many instances circumvented by students studying biomedical problems in a given organ system seeing real patients with problems related to that system to develop the relevant clinical skills.[9,33]

Many basic scientists have experienced difficulty in writing realistic clinical scenarios that lead to fundamental objectives in the basic sciences, particularly in cell and molecular biology.[15] Experience with constructing problems clearly demonstrates that it is sometimes necessary to create problem components that trigger students to consider fundamental basic science concepts in those areas where direct clinical relevance is not seen easily. Jamieson advocates the use of 'scientific scenarios to achieve scientific learning objectives . . . which may still be relevant to clinical life, such as research seminars, hospital laboratories and journal clubs.'[14]

Another factor that enhances integration in problem-based learning is the fact that students are placed in a similar 'psychological environment' to that in which they would apply their learning in future professional life. The psychological environment here refers to the mental context in which daily work is carried out by the professional. The physician is constantly solving problems, mainly concerning the patients or communities he encounters. Furthermore, the physician is looked upon by many as a leader and is expected to deal with problems arising in the healthcare team and those of an administrative nature. Thus it is not an exaggeration to say that the physician lives in a world of problems. Training the future physician in an environment where problem solving is the main mode of learning is likely to result in integrative learning more than other modes, as it is closer to future real life. The concept of psychological environment (though the term was not used as such) is exemplified in a study done by Leyden *et al.*, in which first year medical students learnt about risk factors in coronary heart disease by undergoing a self-change project to modify their own behaviours that contributed to increased risk of disease.[34] Students learnt in an environment in which they were applying their learning to their own health.

Rigidity in 'student set', where problem-solving students follow a routine pattern for all problems, is a deterrent to integrated learning. In one medical school that adopts problem-based tutorials as the main learning experience during a certain phase of the curriculum, in the first meeting students examine the trigger of a given problem very briefly and move rapidly into identifying the disciplines that impinge on the problem. They then ask questions pertaining to each of those disciplines and allocate responsibility to each student for finding the answers to those questions. When they return to the second meeting they share their learning, but since they were each responsible for only one discipline they are often unaware of related concepts from other disciplines. As a result they often do not undertake integrated learning in self-study, and only do so, if at all, when they try to apply their combined learning to the problem in the second meeting. Unfortunately for many the problem is seen as a summation of concepts from different disciplines, rather than the relationships among them. As a result one of the main advantages of problem-based learning is lost.

COMMUNITY-BASED INTEGRATION

A distinction must first be made between the concepts of community-oriented and community-based education, even though one is subsumed by the other. *Community-oriented education* is focused on the healthcare needs of communities, as distinct from those of individuals. *Community-based education* takes place in the environment of the community, rather than in the context of single patients, such as usually takes place in ward-based or clinic-based clinical teaching. Undoubtedly, the ward or the clinic can be thought of as different types of communities. If students learn how to deal with such communities, rather than with the individuals who comprise them, then learning in the ward or the clinic can be classified as community-based learning. However, such is not the usual focus of ward-based and clinic-based learning for medical students, even though it is a desirable aspect of such learning experiences. Community-based learning occurs largely outside the hospital or the clinic, in rural or urban communities, and the students are physically present in these communities when they experience learning. Bruce notes, however, that a 'community-based' approach is community-responsive, community-driven and community-rooted, but is not necessarily community placed.[35] According to the definitions given earlier, such an experience would be classified as community-oriented rather than community-based.

Traditionally, teachers and students become more remote from life situations where education is put to use.[1] The community is one of those situations where the physician puts to use what he learns. Following the principle that learning is more integrated in the context in which that learning is applied, learning in community situations is likely to be more integrative than learning in a lecture theatre. Yet objectives that require the student to relate knowledge to real-life situations are also more integrative.[3] Community-oriented education can take place anywhere, provided the objectives are oriented towards the community. Thus community-oriented learning, even in a lecture theatre, is also likely to be more integrative than learning that is not oriented towards the community, as the objectives of the former require students to relate knowledge to real-life situations in which they would be placed as practising professionals. However, extra-class experiences enable students to relate formal learning to what they do and feel.

The Comprehensive Community Health Project (CCHP) of the University of the Philippines[36] was at one time implemented in a fishing community at Laguna de Bay, an hour's drive from Manila. The project provided for health professions students to live with foster families in the village (*barrio*), experience the daily life of the families with whom they lived and take part in all health-related decisions in the community. The knowledge, skills and attitudes that they gained as a result of this truly integrative experience would undoubtedly have made an indelible impression on their minds and stood them in good stead when they were really called upon to practise in such communities in later professional life. Mayhew suggested that integration could be achieved through fieldwork if judiciously blended with study in the library.[37] Learning in the CCHP depended not so much on library work but on the interchange of experiences each week by the students living with different foster families. For example, a role play that the author was privileged to observe and that made an indelible impression on him was a re-enactment of the dilemma faced by a pregnant woman who was advised by the traditional midwife, on the one hand, and the allopathic physician, on the other. The role play depicted the manner in which the students, who had been placed in that community for a while and had won the confidence of the woman's family, were able to steer a path between these two opposing forces to achieve a happy outcome.

Benor pointed out that learning in real-life settings enhanced the development of attitudes in students.[2] In the absence of adequate opportunities for all students to experience real-life situations, such as that discussed, role play of the real situation experienced by a few would be the second-best option to bring about such development of attitudes. Wilkinson *et al.* found that attitudes to older people were better, among junior medical students in the Christchurch Medical School, after they had early community contact with older people.[38] Students must live in the community for a period of time, as in the CCHP, so that they can observe how members of that community live and get a deeper understanding of their mores. Students from the Wellington Medical School undergo 'cultural immersion' in Maori communities, enabling them to study health problems in their natural context.[39] The WAMI (Washington, Alaska, Montana, Idaho) project set up by the University of Washington School of Medicine in Seattle,[40] now renamed WWAMI with the inclusion of Wyoming,[41] goes a step further in that the spouses of students and residents are encouraged to go to the communities in which students learn, so that they are immersed in the atmosphere of those communities and experience the roles they would be called upon to play if medical practices were established in such areas.

With the growth of community-based learning and the realisation that the traditional tertiary care teaching hospital may not accurately reflect contemporary patterns of disease and healthcare, a trend developed in which large amounts of teaching were shifted from the tertiary care hospital to other settings.[42] However, Katz and Fulop caution us that, if field training centres are to work properly, a functional model for an integrated health centre, where there is coordination among its activities in a manner that its healthcare objectives are more easily reached, must be created.[9] For the physician these activities include the facilitation of the patient's entry into the healthcare system, the provision of preventive healthcare, integrating and ensuring continuity of care and participation in broad activities directed towards the health needs of the population; in short, primary healthcare. These needs may vary from one population to another.

In some situations education must link the medical system to the social and economic needs of the population,[43] as in Beersheva, Israel;[44] in others, as in Australia, the focus may be on the diversity of cultural groups and the teaching of behavioural sciences to deal with such diversity.[45]

Hospital-based education by itself is inadequate for another reason. In this age of escalating healthcare costs, coupled with the relative inadequacy of hospital beds in tertiary care hospitals resulting in shorter hospital stays, the clinical student is inevitably exposed to only a 'snapshot' of a patient's illness, probably at a fairly highly specialised level. However, in the real-life practice of a basic doctor, one has to learn to deal with the entire duration of the illness, and it is mandatory for the medical student to be exposed to continuity of care. This can only be achieved through experiences in primary and secondary care hospitals, general practices and community settings. Oswald *et al.* describe a community-based clinical programme at Cambridge University that enables the student to obtain continuity of contact with patients over a prolonged period integrated with their hospital-based experiences.[46]

The mere revision of course offerings while maintaining a subject-centred format is unlikely to bring medical education closer to the work of a practising physician.[47] The kinds of problems that physicians are faced with in community practice are likely to cut across narrow disciplinary boundaries.[21] If community-oriented medical education is to be integrative, the experiences must be relevant and meaningful to the student in terms of needs, abilities, skills and understanding.[48] The increasing emphasis towards primary healthcare, which has coloured medical education ever since the Alma-Ata Declaration,[49] is unlikely to affect the emphasis on hospital-based care unless curricular reforms look critically at the educational structure that has been ingrained in the institution.[12] Healthcare providers are obsessed with the need for clinical professionalism and continually endeavour to master narrow technical skills, even though clinicians are not trained in, nor are proponents of, community-oriented medical education.[50] Clinical school teachers in medical schools are, by and large, brought up in this tradition, and often unintentionally inculcate such values in their students, who look to them as role models. If community-oriented medical education is to be effective, its teaching should be the concern of all faculty members. Community aspects should be emphasised even by the highly specialised clinician and basic scientist. Community medicine should not be seen as a second-class activity that is the domain only of community medicine faculty. Students must perceive that their role model, the clinician, whom they aim to emulate, holds community-related teaching in high esteem. They must demonstrate how community aspects of care impinge on their daily activities. Only then can true integration take place between clinical and community medicine.

MULTIPROFESSIONAL INTEGRATION

While much confusion exists in the literature of the concept of multiprofessional education in the health sciences, it is here defined as learning experiences arranged for students from two or more health professions together, to enable them to acquire knowledge, skills and attitudes that prepare them to act cooperatively and collaboratively in providing healthcare to the patient and the community. This is distinct from teaching by a single teacher to students from many health professions in a single course, a practice that is commonly followed by basic science departments in the allied health professions, often with the intent of economising on scarce human resources, rather than to develop healthcare teamwork skills in their students.

The concept of multiprofessional integration is based on the axiom that true integrated learning takes place in situations that resemble real life as closely as possible. In the real world the healthcare team functions as a single unit, with each member clearly aware of the role of each of the other members. If learning can take place in such an environment, where health profession students learn together, and at the same time have as one of their objectives the development of an awareness of the roles of each member of the team, then integrated learning takes place in this multiprofessional environment. The main purposes of true multiprofessional learning are to develop abilities in health professional students of working together, sharing information and helping each other learn, to maximise interaction among them so that communication and collaboration in practice could be improved. Reeves *et al.* pointed out that one advantage of health profession students working and learning together in a healthcare team in the ward is that they learn what to expect in the future.[51] The adoption of a more holistic approach fostered by such learning is likely to improve patient outcomes.[52] Barr has emphasised that if students from the different health professions are to understand each others' roles, the learning opportunities afforded them should reflect the reality of healthcare practices in that situation.[53] If multiprofessional integration is to succeed, faculty members from the different health professions should also be prepared and be given time for team building. Furthermore, the learning experiences should be relevant to all categories of students, and should aim at maximising interaction among them.

Another form of multiprofessional integration has been attempted at the University of the Philippines Integrated Health Sciences (IHS) project in Tacloban, Leyte. This programme is designed to train health profession students in primary and secondary rural healthcare through a ladder-type curriculum that permits vertical mobility, in that they can undergo training at increasingly higher levels in the hierarchy of the health team.[54] Thus a student may exit at any level of the curriculum but still be useful to the community according to the level at which he exited. The advantage is that all health profession students learn together and those who exit at the higher levels of the hierarchy are inevitably trained to function at each of the lower levels as well. While the programme adopts a truly multiprofessional approach, one has to question whether it is cost-effective to train, say, a medical graduate to function as a village health worker, a public health nurse and an associate in public health before she graduates as a medical officer.

Many schools have adopted less drastic approaches to inculcate the values espoused by multiprofessional learning. The Faculty of Health Sciences at the University of Linköping in Sweden adopted a multidisciplinary approach, at the commencement of the training programmes for health professionals, in a course entitled 'Man and Society'.[55] Students in laboratory technology, nursing, occupational therapy, medicine, physiotherapy and social service undertake problem-based learning in multiprofessional groups on societal and behavioural science problems.

The School of Medicine at the University of Auckland introduced, in 1984, a lecture-interview programme, which was replaced two years later by a self-directed programme, in which third-year students learn about the skills and knowledge of other health professionals.[56] While this strategy cannot be called multiprofessional learning according to the earlier definition, it attempted to achieve some of the objectives of the latter. At best it informs medical students of the roles of the other members of the healthcare team, and perhaps changes their attitudes to these members, but does not necessarily improve their skills in teamwork. One study indicated that medical students were willing to share responsibility with nurses if they had the perception that they learnt a given topic from nurses during a multidisciplinary course in ambulatory care for diabetic patients.[57] More studies on the impact of multiprofessional courses, in terms of both educational achievement and effects on patient care, are indicated if multiprofessional education is to become an enduringly useful strategy for integration.

INTEGRATION OF THE SCIENCE AND THE ART OF MEDICINE

Organ made the seemingly obvious remark that 'scientific values translated into action without concern for human values can plunge mankind into barbarism'.[58]

The science and art of medicine are closely linked. In spite of this the introduction of the behavioural sciences into the medical curriculum was long delayed, as pointed out in Chapter 2. When ultimately these sciences did appear there seemed to be much confusion at first as to what exactly should be included and when it should be included. A survey undertaken by Gwee in 1978 revealed that, in the early years of introduction of the behavioural sciences, there was much variation in the aims of the courses that were offered to medical students, ranging from the development of communication skills to the management of behavioural disorders.[59] These same differences persist in the medical curriculum of today, though some aims seem to be more uniformly addressed as the trend develops. This section is concerned with the manner in which behavioural science teaching has been integrated into the existing curriculum. Undoubtedly this depends on the nature of the course content. The wide variety of courses precludes consideration of all content areas. Hence the consideration of integration will be confined to two common areas that most schools are increasingly focusing on in their attempts to inculcate humanistic values in their students; namely, communication skills and medical ethics.

There is much overlap between these two areas. For example, one survey found that some medical schools in the United Kingdom regarded medical ethics as part of communication skills training.[60] Yet their importance for similar and dissimilar reasons warrants their separate consideration, either as separate courses or courses interwoven with existing courses.

Communication skills

The pre-eminent place that communication skills hold in the work of a physician mandates their deliberate inculcation in medical students during training. Training in these skills was, however, largely neglected or incidental during the greater part of the last century, as they were overwhelmed by the ever-expanding basic and clinical sciences. When communication skills training was first introduced, separate courses in the earlier years of the curriculum seemed to be the trend. The futility of such efforts without reinforcement during the latter phases of the curriculum soon became evident. The reason for this was similar to that which resulted in the basic sciences being forgotten by the time students reached the clinical years. Separate courses were seen as hurdles to get over before moving on to the more important clinical sciences. Communication skills learnt in isolation were not seen as relevant. If relevance is to be perceived such training must be integrated with existing courses both horizontally and vertically.

A needs assessment at Dalhousie Medical School showed that communication skills training in the early years of the curriculum were not reinforced in clerkship or residency training.[61] As a result of this assessment a programme was developed that integrated communication skills training across the curriculum in the following manner: in Year 1, training in conducting a medical interview; in Year 2, including a communication skills component in each of four problem-based units; and, in the clerkship phase, focusing on consolidating previous skills as well as dealing with communication challenges.

The survey in 26 medical schools in the United Kingdom referred to previously showed that the responsibility for implementing communication skills training was spread across a range of specialisms.[60] The authors surmised that this finding probably reflected a General Medical Council recommendation that communication skills training should be integrated within the overall curriculum.[62] The mere fact that training was undertaken by different specialities does not guarantee, however, that these training components are integrated in any one school. Even if a given school offered a curriculum in which communication skills were dealt with across several departments or course units, integration requires such training to be linked in a manner that students perceive wholeness in what they learn and relevance to their future roles.

Another level of integration in communication skills training is between theoretical and practical components of communication. In the earlier years many health professional schools offered communication skills training in the form of a series of didactic lectures on the communication process. These lectures laid down the theoretical basis of effective communication and discussed problems that could arise in the communication process at a theoretical level, but did not offer the student opportunities to practise communication using this theoretical base. This deficiency was evident to the author in an evaluative study undertaken to determine deficiencies in training of health workers for family healthcare in a South East Asian country.[63] The theoretical courses on communication had little effect on the actual communication patterns adopted by the health workers. The survey referred to found that 15 of the 26 British medical schools integrated theoretical and practical components of communication skills training.[60] Those schools in which the responsibility for teaching communication was entrusted to departments of behavioural science were more likely to use role play as a method of teaching. Role play enabled effective integration of theory and practice, and proved to be an effective way of enhancing attitudes and communication skills. Nevertheless, reinforcement of these skills through supervised practice in real situations such as in the ward, the clinic and the community is essential. Evans *et al.* found that students acquire the most effective interview skills when interacting with patients during their clinical training,[64] while Orbell and Abraham, evaluating a community interview scheme for preclinical medical students, concluded that they valued the opportunity to interview real people to develop their communication skills.[65]

An important issue to consider is who should be responsible for teaching communication skills. A more recent survey by Hargie *et al.* of 21 of the 33 medical schools in the United Kingdom, to whom questionnaires were administered, showed that in 86% of them a dedicated staff member, usually a psychologist, had responsibility for coordinating such teaching throughout the curriculum.[66] While such coordination is a desirable practice to ensure continuity of training, teaching should be the responsibility of all the teachers in the school, in particular the clinical teachers, who serve as the most potent role models in the school for the vast majority of students. Depending on the degree of importance the former attach to communication, they may serve as good or poor role models. Although a survey of faculty attitudes towards communication at Dalhousie University indicated that clinical teachers had a positive attitude,[68] one must be careful in interpreting actual behaviours from responses to attitude questionnaires. The most important factor shaping student attitudes is the overt expression, observed by the students, of clinicians' attitudes through their behaviours in their daily interactions with patients and other members of the healthcare team. Herein is the importance for training of integrating good communication practices in real-life situations. Thus it would be ideal if a core team of behaviourists and clinicians 'has central responsibility for communication skills training, coordinating tutors variously involved throughout the curriculum',[60] integrating such training both horizontally and vertically. Whitehouse, whose previous survey in UK schools found a reported lack of integration among departments, recommends a core group of 'highly trained educators drawn from behavioural science, medicine and education . . . professionally committed to communication skills teaching and assessment . . . integrated with the informal reinforcement of such teaching . . . in clinical practice'.[68]

Medical ethics

While from the time of Hippocrates the need for inculcating ethical principles and the ideals of the profession of medicine in the training of the medical student has been recognised, many factors led to the trend of including special courses in medical ethics in the undergraduate curriculum. These factors have been outlined in an editorial on the teaching of medical ethics in medical schools by Al-Mahroos and Bandaranayake.[69] The Nuremberg trials of 1947, scientific advances in medicine with an associated loss of the humane side of the profession, ethical dilemmas in research, rapid advances in the field of genetics and the increasing demystification of the profession, hastened by the growth of the internet, with an accompanying increase in the frequency of medical litigation, are but some of these factors that led to this trend. In this section we will consider the manner in which courses in medical ethics have been integrated into the undergraduate medical curriculum.

Seedhouse states that there cannot be a discipline of medical ethics as it has 'no definitive core of knowledge or theory and is parasitic on moral philosophy and clinical practice', and one cannot 'distinguish ethical from non-ethical problems in the medical care of living beings'.[70] He argues that any intervention undertaken by a doctor has a bearing on ethics, but the correct ethical procedure to follow varies with the nature of the intervention and the circumstances under which that intervention occurs. It is thus apparent that ethical practices have to be inculcated in students in the context of care administered to individual patients, rather than as separate theoretical courses. Thus medical ethics must necessarily be integrated with other parts of the undergraduate curriculum. Instead of adding yet another speciality to the overcrowded curriculum, he advocates encouraging 'students to think critically, drawing on as much relevant theory and evidence as possible, in order to resolve difficulties'[70] that may arise in interventions. This task can be carried out by generalists rather than by specialists in medical ethics.

In keeping with this argument, Babapulle states that one of the deficiencies in the teaching of medical ethics is that often an ethical rule is emphasised first, followed by the application of the rule to a given situation, while 'the rule ethic may be inappropriate under certain circumstances, for which a "situation ethic" may be more appropriate'.[71] He states that it is necessary to expose students to the use of ethical principles in forming judgements in different situations. This is, in fact, the essence of vertical integration, and the ethical principles so learnt are likely to be more appreciated, and perhaps better retained, by students, as they can see their relevance to future practice.

While observing a problem-based tutorial for a group of senior medical students in an American medical school, the author was impressed by the manner in which the students were allowed by the facilitator to digress from the stipulated objectives of the neurological problem, to a prolonged discussion of the ethical aspects of the situation. He realised that much learning was taking place in the students, even though such learning was not intended from the problem. When the scheduled tutorial time ran out without the intended objectives being achieved, he distributed the latter to the students, requesting them to undertake self-directed learning later. The facilitator demonstrated his true role in this episode, and undoubtedly the students realised the importance of the ethical aspects of the problem through their discussion.

Many are the examples cited in the literature of practical exercises that help to bridge the gap between the classroom and actual clinical practice.[72] A comparison of ethics programmes in two medical schools in the Netherlands led to the conclusion that a powerful model for clinical ethics teaching would be a combination of a theoretical framework leading to a method for case analysis and interpretation, and the application of this method using relevant cases, undertaken by a team of an ethicist and a clinician.[73]

It is obvious that, if such learning experiences are to be successful, not only must clinical psychologists collaborate effectively with clinical colleagues in exposing students to the practical implications of psychological theories[74] but also students must actually see their clinical teachers apply these theories through practice in their daily work. As will be pointed out in Chapter 6, however, these efforts will not be effective unless due emphasis is placed on medical ethics in student assessment in a manner that calls upon students not only to display their knowledge but also to apply that knowledge in clinical situations.[75]

KEY POINTS

- Many teachers continue to train students as though they were training clones of their own speciality.
- The integrative nature of specific learning objectives lies in their ability to call upon critical thinking based on knowledge from related disciplines or courses.
- Integration does not take place because of any particular method or curricular organisation unless it engages the student in integrative activity.

- Problem-based learning has the potential to reach the acme of integration, but integrated learning will only take place if students are given the opportunity, and are required, to undertake linking among disciplines.
- No one discipline can isolate itself from the others as knowledge used in one is both dependent and influential on the others.
- Basic sciences should be integrated with clinical sciences in both preclinical and clinical phases of the curriculum.
- If community-oriented medical education is to be effective for integrated learning, its teaching should be the concern of all faculty members in the school.
- When health profession students learn together to develop awareness of each others' roles in the healthcare team, integrated learning takes place in a multiprofessional environment.
- If communication skills training is to be perceived as relevant it must be integrated with established courses.
- Students should be exposed to the use of ethical principles in forming judgements in different clinical and community settings.

REFERENCES

1 Dressel PL. The meaning and significance of integration. In: Henry NB, editor. *The Integration of Educational Experiences*, 57th Yearbook of the National Society for the Study of Education, Part III. Chicago, IL: University of Chicago Press; 1958, Chapter I, pp. 3–25 and Chapter XII, pp. 251–63.

2 Benor DE. Interdisciplinary integration in medical education: theory and method. *Med Educ*. 1982; **16**: 355–61.

3 Pace CR. Educational objectives. In: Henry NB, editor. *The Integration of Educational Experiences*, op. cit., Chapter IV, pp. 69–83.

4 Koestler A. *The Act of Creation*. London: Penguin; 1964. p. 13.

5 Guilbert J-J. 'Coveritis': an acute and chronic faculty disease. *Educação Medica*. 1995; **6**: 2–7.

6 Abrahamson S. Diseases of the curriculum. *J Med Educ*. 1978; **53**: 951–7.

7 Rodin AE, Taylor JD, Hnatko SI, *et al*. The correlative laboratory as a method for the integrated teaching of medicine. *J Med Educ*. 1964; **39**: 540–4.

8 Spilman E. The multidisciplinary laboratories. *J Med Educ* 1958; **33**: 168–74.

9 Katz J, Fulop T. Personnel for health care: case studies of educational programmes. *Public Health Pap*. 1978; **70**: 1–260.

10 Ganguly PK, Chakravarty M, Latif NA, *et al*. Teaching of anatomy in a problem-based curriculum at the Arabian Gulf University: the new face of the museum. *Clin Anat*. 2003; **16**: 256–61.

11 Goodlad JI. Illustrative programs and procedures in elementary schools.

In: Henry NB, editor. *The Integration of Educational Experiences*, op. cit., Chapter IX, pages 173–93.

12 Armstrong D. The structure of medical education. *Med Educ.* 1977; **11**, 244–8.

13 Bloom BS. Ideas, problems and methods of inquiry. In: Henry NB, editor. *The Integration of Educational Experiences*, op. cit., Chapter V, pp. 84–104.

14 Jamieson S. Cell and molecular biology in the medical curriculum. *Med Educ.* 2001; **35**: 83–7.

15 Gellhorn A, Scheuer R. The experiment in medical education at the City College of New York. *J Med Educ.* 1978; **53**: 574–82.

16 Hayter CR. Physics for physicians: integrating science into the medical curriculum, 1910–1950. *Acad Med.* 1996; **71**: 1211–17.

17 Kilminster SM, Delmotte A, Frith H, *et al.* Teaching in the new NHS: the specialised ward based teacher. *Med Educ.* 2001; **35**: 437–43.

18 Stout RW, Irwin WG. Integrated medical student teaching. *Med Educ.* 1982; **16**: 143–6.

19 Wallace P, Berlin A, Murray E, *et al.* CeMENT: evaluation of a regional development programme integrating hospital and general practice clinical training for medical undergraduates. *Med Educ.* 2001; **35**: 160–6.

20 Krathwohl DR. The psychological bases for integration. In: Henry NB, editor. *The Integration of Educational Experiences*, op. cit., Chapter III, pp. 43–65.

21 Tyler RW. Curriculum organization. In: Henry NB, editor. *The Integration of Educational Experiences*, op. cit., Chapter VI, pp. 105–25.

22 Christie RV. Trends in medical education. *J Med Educ.* 1963; **38**: 662–6.

23 Basset LW, Squire LF. Anatomy instruction by radiologists. *Invest Radiol.* 1985; **20**: 1008–10.

24 Vieira JE, do Patrocinio Tenório Nune M, de Arruda Martins M. Directing student response to early patient contact by questionnaire. *Med Educ.* 2003; **37**: 119–25.

25 Kachur EK. Commentary. *Med Educ.* 2003; **37**: 88–9.

26 MacLeod RD, Parkin C, Pullon S, *et al.* Early clinical exposure to people who are dying. *Med Educ.* 2003; **37**: 51–8.

27 Abu-Hijleh MF, Chakravarty M, Hamdy H. Clinical anatomy in the clerkship phase of a problem-based medical curriculum. *Med Educ.* 2004; **38**: 551.

28 Heylings DJA. Anatomy 1999–2000: the curriculum, who teaches it and how? *Med Educ.* 2002; **36**: 702–10.

29 Prince KJ, van Mameren H, Hylkema N, *et al.* Does problem-based learning lead to deficiencies in basic science knowledge? An empirical case on anatomy. *Med Educ.* 2003; **37**: 15–21.

30 Maudsley G. The limits of tutors' comfort zones with four integrated knowledge themes in a problem-based undergraduate medical curriculum (Interview study). *Med Educ.* 2003; **37**: 417–23.

31 Goldie J, Schwartz L, McConnachie A, *et al.* The impact of three years' ethics

teaching, in an integrated medical curriculum, on students' proposed behaviour on meeting ethical dilemmas. *Med Educ.* 2002; **36**: 489–97.

32 Schmidt HG. Problem-based learning: rationale and description. *Med Educ.* 1983; **17**: 11–16.

33 Hamdy H, Greally M, Grant IN, *et al.* Professional skills programme in a problem-based learning curriculum: experience at the College of Medicine & Medical Sciences, Arabian Gulf University. *Med Teach.* 2001; **23**: 214–16.

34 Leyden D, Cullinane EM, Wincze J, *et al.* Teaching behavioural medicine using individual coronary heart disease risk factors. *Prev Med.* 1987; **16**: 269–73.

35 Bruce TA. Medical education in community sites (Editorial). *Med Educ.* 1996; **30**: 81–2.

36 Hitalia MLA. The community as a learning environment. In: Bandaranayake R, editor. *Trends in Curricula II.* Sydney: University of New South Wales Press; 1980. pp. 1–14.

37 Mayhew LB. Illustrative courses and programs in colleges and universities. In: Henry NB, editor. *The Integration of Educational Experiences*, op. cit., Chapter XI, pp. 218–48.

38 Wilkinson TJ, Gower S, Sainsbury R. The earlier, the better: the effect of early community contact on the attitudes of medical students to older people. *Med Educ.* 2002; **36**: 540–2.

39 Dowel A, Crampton P, Parkin C. The first sunrise: an experience of cultural immersion and community health needs assessment by undergraduate medical students in New Zealand. *Med Educ.* 2001; **35**: 242–9.

40 Schwarz MR, Flahault D. The WAMI programme, University of Washington School of Medicine, Seattle, WA, United States of America: decentralizing medical education. *Public Health Pap.* 1978; **70**: 229–50.

41 Schwarz MR. The WAMI Program: 25 years later. *Med Teach.* 2004; **26**: 211–14.

42 Wallace P, Berlin A, Murray E, *et al.* CeMENT: evaluation of a regional development programme integrating hospital and general practice clinical teaching for medical undergraduates. *Med Educ.* 2001; **35**: 160–6.

43 Ramalingaswami V. Medical education: how is change to come about? *Med Educ.* 1989; **23**: 328–32.

44 Prywes M. The Beersheva experience: a new centre for health sciences in the Negev, Israel. *Med Educ.* 1978; **12** (Suppl.): S10–11.

45 Klein D. Teaching the behavioural sciences to medical students: some observations on Australia. *Med J Aust.* 1976; **1**: 536–8.

46 Oswald N, Alderson T, Jones S. Evaluating primary care as a base for medical education: the report of the Cambridge Community-based Clinical Course. *Med Educ.* 2001; **35**: 782–8.

47 McGaghie WC, Miller GE, Sajid AW, *et al.* Competency-based curriculum development in medical education: an introduction. *Public Health Pap.* 1978; **68**: 11–91.

48 Churchill R, Rothman P. Extraclass experiences. In: Henry NB, editor. *The Integration of Educational Experiences*, op. cit., Chapter VII, pp. 126–42.

49 World Health Organization. *Global Strategy of Health for All by the Year 2001*, Series No. 3. Geneva: World Health Organization; 1981.

50 Connor LH, Higginbotham N. An integrated sociocultural curriculum for community medicine in Bali, Indonesia. *Soc Sci Med.* 1986; **23**: 673–82.

51 Reeves S, Freeth D, McCrorie P, *et al.* 'It teaches you what to expect in future . . .': interprofessional learning on a training ward for medical, nursing, occupational therapy and physiotherapy students. *Med Educ.* 2002; **36**: 337–44.

52 Eva KW. Teamwork during education: the whole is not always greater than the sum of the parts. *Med Educ.* 2002; **36**: 314–16.

53 Barr H. Ends and means in interprofessional education: towards a typology. *Educ Health (Abingdon).* 1996; **9**: 341–52.

54 Abarquez LF. Increasing emphasis on community and preventive medicine. In: Bandaranayake R, editor. *Trends in Curricula.* Sydney: University of New South Wales Press; 1979, pp. 29–44.

55 Bergdahl B, Koch M, Ludvigsson J, *et al.* The Linköping medical programme: a curriculum for student-centered learning. *Annals of Community-Oriented Education.* 1994; **7**: 107–19.

56 Grant V. Teaching medical students about other health professionals: an experiment in self-directed learning. *Med Teach,* 1987; **9**: 271–4.

57 Lorenz RA, Pichert JW. Impact of interprofessional training on medical students' willingness to accept clinical responsibility. *Med Educ.* 1986; **20**: 195–200.

58 Organ TW. Integration in higher education. *J Higher Educ.* 1955; **26**: 180–6.

59 Gwee M. The introduction of social and behavioural sciences into the medical curriculum. In: Bandaranayake R, editor. *Trends in Curricula,* op. cit., p. 11.

60 Hargie O, Dickson D, Boohan M, *et al.* A survey of communication skills training in UK schools of medicine: present practices and prospective proposals. *Med Educ.* 1998; **32**: 25–34.

61 Laidlaw TS, MacLeod H, Kaufman DM, *et al.* Implementing a communication skills programme in medical school: needs assessment and programme change. *Med Educ.* 2002; **36**: 115–24.

62 General Medical Council. *Tomorrow's Doctors: recommendations on undergraduate medical education.* London: General Medical Council; 1993.

63 Bandaranayake RC, Singh PJ. Using tracers to link health services to training through evaluation. *Med Educ.* 1993; **27**: 509–17.

64 Evans BJ, Sweet B, Coman GJ. Behavioural assessment of the effectiveness of a communication programme for medical students. *Med Educ.* 1993; **27**: 344–50.

65 Orbell S, Abraham C. Behavioural sciences and the real world: report of a community interview scheme for medical students. *Med Educ.* 1993; **27**: 218–28.

66 Hargie O, Boohan M, McCoy M, *et al.* Current trends in Communication Skills training in UK schools of medicine. *Med Teach.* 2010; **32**: 385–91.

67 Langille DB, Kaufman DM, Laidlaw TA, *et al.* Faculty attitudes towards medical communication and their perceptions of students' communication skills training at Dalhousie University. *Med Educ.* 2001; **35**: 548–54.

68 Whitehouse CR. The teaching of communication skills in United Kingdom medical schools. *Med Educ.* 1991; **25**: 311–18.

69 Al-Mahroos F, Bandaranayake R. Teaching medical ethics in medical schools (Editorial). *Ann Saudi Med.* 2003; **23**: 1–5.

70 Seedhouse D. Against medical ethics: a philosopher's view (Editorial). *Med Edu.* 1991; **25**: 280–2.

71 Babapulle CJ. Teaching of medical ethics in Sri Lanka. *Med Educ.* 1992; **26**: 185–9.

72 Mitchell KR, Lovat TJ, Myser CM. Teaching bioethics to medical students: the Newcastle experience. *Med Educ.* 1992; **26**: 290–300.

73 ten Have HA. Ethics in the clinic: a comparison of two Dutch teaching programmes. *Med Educ.* 1995; **29**: 34–8.

74 Kent GG. The role of psychology in the teaching of medical ethics: the example of informed consent. *Med Educ.* 1994; **28**: 126–31.

75 Myser C, Kerridge III, Mitchell KR. Ethical reasoning and decision-making in the clinical setting: assessing the process. *Med Educ.* 1995; **29**: 29–33.

CHAPTER 5

Advantages and disadvantages of curriculum integration

The attempts at integration reviewed in the previous chapter have also indicated many of the advantages associated with integrated curricula. This chapter will critically examine these and other advantages and disadvantages.

Advantages and disadvantages of integrated curricula accrue to both the student and the teacher. These must be examined in relation to the role that each is called upon to play. The contribution that these roles make to society must be the final determinant of whether a particular characteristic of an integrated curriculum is an advantage or a disadvantage, and the extent to which it is so. In making judgements about these characteristics one must be cautious to separate intentions from outcomes. For example, a problem-based curriculum may have very laudable intentions for student learning, but the actual outcomes will depend very much on how the intentions are translated to practice, both by the student and by the teacher.

ADVANTAGES TO THE STUDENT

The medical student's role is to acquire such knowledge, skills and attitudes as would make her a caring and skilled professional for supervised practice, and as a foundation for independent practice with further training in a given field of endeavour.

One of the major problems experienced by the medical student is the retention of information that she has acquired over a long period of study. Retention of information depends on many factors. Two of the most important are meaningfulness and relevance. In Chapter 1 the difference between these two concepts was explained. In summary, meaningfulness is the extent to which new learning fits with the learner's existing learning; relevance is the extent to which new learning is perceived by the learner as useful to her envisaged role. As any form of integration attempts to make meaningful wholes out of constituent parts, and as reality is the substrate of integration, integrative learning is likely to be more meaningful than piecemeal learning. If the learner can link several ideas and shape them into a single idea by making links among them, she would acquire greater depth of meaning and be able to recall those ideas better and for a longer period.[1] Retention is aided by organisation of ideas, and organisation is central to integration, as integration of ideas helps the learner to organise them into a smaller number of packages, each of which is richer by itself.[1] Similarly, organisation of experiences reduces a large number of separate experiences into a smaller number of groups.[2] Recall of one experience would then facilitate recall of the whole group to which that experience belongs. When two separate experiences are grouped together, they may take on added significance, stimulating creativity through the process of 'bisociation', referred to in Chapter 4. If the student who learns some information in one classroom is able to link it to what she learns in another (i.e. to integrate) retention is enhanced. Rosse showed that students who followed an early integrated organ-systems course had significantly better knowledge on that course at the point of graduation than those who followed a non-integrated course.[3] However, it is essential that this linking must be undertaken by the student rather than the teacher if this advantage is to accrue. While linking by the teacher undoubtedly facilitates retention, it is most effective if the integration is undertaken by the student. The student who consciously seeks meaningful relationships between isolated bits of information has gone a long way towards developing skills of self-directed learning.[2]

Schmidt identified three major elements in the process of problem-based learning: activation, where existing knowledge is used to understand and structure new information; encoding, if the learning situation is close to the application of that learning; and elaboration, where opportunities are provided, through discussion and questioning, to understand the newly acquired information. Activation promotes understanding, encoding facilitates transfer and elaboration aids retention.[4]

Relevance aids retention of information by increasing motivation to learn as well as by its potential for the learner to make meaningful applications of what is learnt as learning progresses. Integration, particularly vertical integration, of learning increases relevance as it provides opportunities for the learner to apply theoretical learning to practical situations. The education of the medical student is brought closer to the work of the practitioner.[5] When junior medical students at the University of Hong Kong were exposed to clinical skills within an integrated systems-based course with problem-based learning, one of the main advantages pointed out by them was that they were able to 'see the real thing'.[6] Colliver points out that 'almost all of clinical education occurs in the contextually relevant process of patient care'.[7]

However, in most discipline-based curricula this exposure either comes long after students are exposed to the basic science foundations of that care or the theoretical basis of illness is not synchronised with its practical application in the context of patients and the community. The advantage of vertical integration is that the relevance of what is learnt is seen immediately after it is learnt, thereby increasing motivation, facilitating relevance and aiding transfer to novel situations when the need arises.

Marton and Säljö identified two basic approaches to learning: deep learning, which requires the learner to understand what is learnt, and surface learning, where facts and concepts are memorised without noting the underlying structure and principles.[8] Integration enhances deep learning because it calls upon the learner to establish links. In order to do so, understanding must first have taken place. The learner who undertakes deep learning attempts to integrate new ideas and facts with what he already knows. The outcome of such learning is a deeper understanding of the learning task.[9] While horizontally integrated learning by itself makes it imperative for the learner to undertake deep learning, vertical integration enhances it further, as application of theoretical facts to practical situations, such as the clinical encounter, requires the establishment of deeper meaningful links. As problem-based learning requires the learner to draw associations between existing learning and the problems presented in the triggers, and to acquire that learning that does not exist but is requisite for the solution of the problem, it should also enhance deep learning. However, as pointed out, in some situations where problem-based learning is implemented, this major advantage is lost if the learner undertakes non-integrative learning after the initial exposure to the problem.

Integration develops the creative thinking of the student if it encourages him to form his own opinions and insights about issues of importance to him.[10] The development of this attribute is dependent on the nature of the learning experiences to which he is exposed. If the integrative experience is teacher-dominated, creativity is suppressed even though integration is enhanced. As creative thinking is a central attribute of the physician and a major educational objective of medical education,[11] opportunities to develop this attribute must be included in any integrated programme.

Another practical advantage of integration is the reduction of redundancy. This is particularly important in an era of knowledge explosion, where it is impossible for the medical student to master all the knowledge that is expected of him. The duplication of knowledge, which is inevitable in a programme where there is no collaboration among teachers planning and implementing it for the same students, is often unnecessary and at the expense of, perhaps, more useful information. This is not to say that reinforcement of knowledge is unnecessary. On the other hand, it is mandatory if retention is to be facilitated. However, there is a difference between reinforcement and repetition. The former can be achieved by calling upon the student to apply knowledge he has acquired to new situations that are encountered along the path to professional training. Gross anatomy is a case in point. For a long time, as a cornerstone of medical practice, it had enjoyed the privilege of inordinate curriculum time, during which students learnt this important subject in various ways. As the curriculum in the different disciplines was often not coordinated, physiology, for example, was learnt in virtually total isolation from gross anatomy. However, the physiologist often repeated, albeit in an abbreviated form, the gross anatomy of the part of the body that was the focus of the teaching of function, as it was critical to the understanding of function. This was repeated in pathology, surgery and so on, mostly because the gross anatomy learnt in isolation had been largely forgotten by the student. Heylings has challenged anatomists to develop new approaches to the teaching of gross anatomy through vertical integration of the subject with clinical sciences, if it is to regain its status.[12] When collaboration does exist in planning through such means as interdisciplinary committees, as is mandatory in a truly integrated programme, a balanced educational programme would result, without the usual conflicts for curriculum time, which is a common feature of discipline-based programmes.[13]

The advantages of multidisciplinary integration have already been alluded to. All participants in the multidisciplinary learning process develop broader perspectives regarding one another's professions, particularly their values, purposes and abilities.[14] As a result these programmes provide a good platform for preparing the future practitioner.

ADVANTAGES TO THE TEACHER

The greatest advantage of an integrated curriculum to the teacher is that it encourages faculty development. As teachers become aware of one another's contributions, through collaborative planning and implementation, they develop mutual respect for colleagues, in stark contrast to the departmental isolation they usually experience in a discipline-based curriculum. They come to realise that many of the problems they experience are common, and attempts to find joint solutions to those problems are more likely to be successful. Through observation they learn about one another's teaching styles and preparation techniques, and they grow intellectually from the learning they gain from listening to their colleagues in other disciplines.[15] In vertical integration, basic scientists and clinical faculty interact to an extent that the former get a broader perspective of their discipline through clinical application,[16] while the scientific attitude adopted by the latter may be enhanced.[17] Such close relationships not only enhance teaching but also may lead to more collaborative research projects.[12] An added advantage of integrated curricula, which include integrated assessment, is that the cooperation among teachers from different disciplines in constructing and scoring assessments leads to improved assessment skills on the part of the teacher.[18]

In a clinical teaching programme where horizontal integration was attempted between hospital and general practice training, Wallace *et al.* found that the morale of the general practice tutors was raised and their confidence and skills improved, while the students who participated in the programme were able to obtain a more balanced view of the continuity of care.[19] At a time when community practitioners are increasingly being called upon to participate in teaching medical students, encouraging and developing this valuable resource would go a long way to sharing the burden of teaching medical students in busy tertiary care teaching hospitals.

DISADVANTAGES TO THE TEACHER AND TO THE STUDENT

Several disadvantages of integrated curricula have been identified in the literature. A careful examination of each of these disadvantages reveals that they are more perceived than real. Many have arisen from the apprehension that accompanies attempts at bringing about such a drastic change in a discipline-based system that has stood the test of time over many decades. Some have resulted from misunderstanding of the concept of integration, or inadequate attention to its planning and implementation. Nevertheless, it is worth reviewing these disadvantages, as ignoring them may create barriers to effective implementation of an integrated curriculum.

Two major disadvantages that have been identified are the difficulty of implementing integration and the amount of time that teachers have to devote to teaching activities if such a curriculum is introduced. The latter is of particular importance as universities are increasingly demanding from teachers research productivity and procurement of research funding, in the face of the diminishing academic dollar.

Teachers in medical school are trained along strict disciplinary lines, and practise their specialities throughout their professional life. The major difficulty arises from the fact that a specialist is called upon to train a student to be a generalist. The specialist has difficulty getting out of his cocoon of specialisation, which he practises on a daily basis. A considerable amount of effort is required if he is to be able to relate material from a number of different fields to his own. The broader the field the more is the potential for integration with other fields and the more difficult it is for him. The teacher who is undertaking research in a very narrow field, such as, say, neurosecretion in the hypothalamus, is either knowledgeable or willing to acquire knowledge in all aspects of that field irrespective of the discipline he belongs to. Thus he must know about the macroscopic structure, microscopic structure, development and function of the hypothalamus, the chemistry of neurosecretion, derangements of neurosecretory function and their effects on the body. He would willingly undertake study in these other fields within that narrow area, as it is essential for his research. Presumably, if he were called upon to teach students in that narrow area, he would be able to do so without much difficulty, as he possesses versatility in knowledge in that area. However, when he is called upon to undertake teaching in many such areas he experiences difficulty. As stated by Becher,

> people, who in one part of their lives [*research*] have to school themselves to
> work in a highly focused way within a confined epistemological space, are

required in another part of their lives [*teaching*] to communicate a broad understanding of their subject fields.[20]

This difficulty is experienced both in preparation for teaching and in its implementation. The specialist forgets, however, that the depth to which each of these disciplines has to be learnt by the medical student is such that it would permit the latter to practise, knowledgeably, as a generalist physician who has the potential to specialise, subsequently, in the discipline of his choice. Senior faculty in academic clinical departments often complain about the ability of the general practitioner to tutor students in problem-based courses, or to undertake clinical teaching as effectively as their clinical colleagues in the teaching hospital.[19] However, as the nature of the tertiary care hospital changes, with shorter hospital stays and more discrimination in the nature of patients admitted to them than was the case earlier, it is becoming increasingly important for the general practitioner to participate in the teaching activities of the medical school, to optimise the chances of students experiencing continuity of patient care, particularly in relation to the common conditions that he is likely to encounter as a basic doctor.

A different type of difficulty arises for teachers who are called upon to teach in a multiprofessional setting; namely, the challenge of developing course material that is relevant and of interest to all students. If, say, a medical student is trained to work in a healthcare team, then the teacher of that student must be aware of the roles of the other members of that team. Hence it would be necessary for that teacher to direct her teaching in terms of the team rather than the individual. In this way she could make her teaching relevant and interesting to all the students who aspire to be members of that team.

One of the biggest disadvantages of integrated curricula is said to be that it is costly in terms of faculty time.[21,13] If this disadvantage is examined carefully it becomes evident that more time is required for planning, both for teaching and for student assessment in an integrated curriculum, rather than for actual implementation of that teaching and assessment. A review of the Association of American Medical Colleges Directory of Medical Schools for 1980–81, undertaken by the author many years ago, at a time when integrated curricula were being implemented in a few medical schools, revealed that there was no significant difference in the average amounts of time reported to have been devoted to teaching between integrated and discipline-based programmes in North American medical schools.[22] Undoubtedly teachers involved in an integrated curriculum would spend much time in interdisciplinary meetings for planning such programmes. This was very evident to the author during a consultancy in a problem-based curriculum, where informal and formal discussion among teachers occupied a significant portion of their time, much more so than in a discipline-based curriculum. However, this is because, in the latter, teachers who have over the years been responsible for certain parts of the curriculum undertake very little planning themselves, repeating what they have taught in previous years, often without any revision. The positive effects of interdisciplinary meetings have already been referred to here. If discipline-based curricula were subjected to the constant review and replanning that they deserve, avoiding entrenchment and gradual loss of touch with reality, then perhaps the difference in planning time would not be so great. In fact the same fate could befall an integrated curriculum if it is not kept under constant review.[23]

Does an integrated curriculum result in less knowledge of the total subject matter in a given discipline than in a discipline-based curriculum? Gaps in the knowledge of a subject in an integrated curriculum have been of concern to educators for a long time. Capehart pointed out that a danger of the problem-solving approach is that important aspects of knowledge may be omitted and superficial solutions to the problem obtained.[24] This is usually overcome in a problem-based curriculum by the deliberate identification of these important areas related to a given problem, and construction of triggers in such a manner as to lead students to the identification of these areas. Students in such programmes are then required to ensure that they either possess the knowledge or acquire it through the learning needs identified during the problem-solving session. Frequent complaints have been heard that 'integration reduces the high standard of knowledge' or that it 'would reduce knowledge of important aspects of a subject as the amount of information memorised is reduced'.[13]

Matrices have been developed in some schools to indicate the extent to which the 'ground is covered' by students in a course of studies and the extent to which each discipline is represented in the curriculum. Prince *et al.* found that problem-based learning did not result in a lower level of anatomical knowledge than more traditional approaches.[25] Many schools that adopt an integrated curriculum have shown a reluctance to give up regional anatomy courses on the basis that there is something to be gained from a regional approach.[12] Certain subjects do have an internal logic, which can be more easily displayed to the student through subject-specific courses. While such courses are easier for the teacher in a given discipline to implement, the issue is whether they are necessarily better for student learning. Certainly they may be more efficient in that they would involve less effort and time. They are unlikely to be more effective, though, if effectiveness is determined by the extent to which knowledge gained is retained and applied. Students, accustomed as they are to subject-centred teaching, display a high level of anxiety in an integrated curriculum, at least initially, when they are uncertain as to the width and depth of a subject they are expected to master. This is not easily apparent to them in integrated curricula. Furthermore, as will be shown later, this concern is exacerbated when assessment procedures, such as national licensing examinations, adopt a discipline-based approach to assessment.

As Chrisman pointed out in relation to pre-university education, the major problem with integrated programmes is an attitudinal one, as teachers see integration as unjustifiably trespassing on territory that they consider their personal property.[26] Territoriality continues to be a major problem with integrated curricula in university education as well. A teacher who is interested in student learning, however, should welcome reinforcement of his teaching from any source, even outside his territory. The reluctance that is evident even today of some departments of anatomy to give up timetable hours, which they have for long considered their own for time-consuming activities such as cadaver dissection, stems mostly from an apprehension that other disciplines erode into their time, even if it can be shown that such time may be used more fruitfully in other endeavours. Time in the curriculum continues to be a symbol of power of any given discipline, and faculty continue to spend large amounts of time in planning meetings justifying their need for increasing amounts of time for their respective disciplines. Teaching time may also be directly proportional to budgetary allocations to departments in some schools.

The importance of integrated learning over integrated teaching has been emphasised many times. Some teachers argue that integration of knowledge should be left to the student, and that a teacher who attempts to do so for the student resorts to 'spoon-feeding' the latter (*see* Case Study 1 in Chapter 9). Undoubtedly the teacher cannot, and should not, do all the integration for the student. However, the teacher can encourage integration by students by planning activities that require the student to undertake integrated learning.[10] Krathwohl noted that helping a child who attempts integrative behaviour would increase his self-concept and he is likely to be encouraged by success to undertake such behaviour in the future.[1] If many schools do not promote such activities in the child, it is all the more important for universities to promote and encourage such behaviour as preparation for future professional life. Integration is too important an outcome to be left to chance. The activities that the teacher plans and implements in class would determine the readiness of the learner to integrate. As will be shown in Chapter 6, the manner in which assessment of learning is undertaken will be critical to the extent to which the student undertakes integrated learning. Thus it is the teacher's duty to plan and implement activities that encourage integrated learning, rather than present a neatly integrated package for the student to passively imbibe.

Integrated curricula may not afford students opportunities to delve deeply into a particular discipline of interest. Many students discover their career interest through such opportunities afforded to them during the curriculum. One advantage of incorporating elective components in the curriculum is that they afford students such opportunities. However, an integrated curriculum does give the interested student an opportunity to delve deeply into a particular topic of interest from the viewpoint of all the disciplines that impinge on it.

Another difficulty in student assessment arises when a discipline-centred curriculum attempts to change over to an integrated curriculum, either wholly or in a part of it. Assessment in such a school is usually discipline-based. A student who is strong in one discipline and weak in another usually has the opportunity to pass the former and resit an examination in the latter, if a minimum score has been obtained in it. When the boundaries among disciplines become blurred in integrated assessment, problems are created for decision-making with regard to such a student, as she may be called upon to repeat a subject in which she has demonstrated competence. As discussed in Chapter 6, this is the reason why pass–fail decisions in an integrated curriculum should not be determined discipline-wise but module-wise, when the curriculum consists of integrated modules, each of which is an entity by itself.

From this discussion it is obvious that the advantages of an integrated curriculum far outweigh its disadvantages. However, in planning such a curriculum, the teacher must be acutely aware that what is most important is for the student to undertake integrated learning and should therefore incorporate those activities that promote such learning.

KEY POINTS

- Integrated learning aids retention as it is meaningful and relevant.
- Integration enhances deep learning as it calls upon the student to establish links.
- Integration develops creative thinking as it encourages the student to form her own opinions about issues of importance to her.
- Repetition of content is reduced in an integrated curriculum, while reinforcement of learning is enhanced.
- An integrated curriculum promotes faculty development as teachers become aware of one another's contributions.
- In an integrated curriculum, teachers spend more time in planning, but not necessarily in implementing the plan.
- Teachers who are immersed in their own speciality may have difficulty at first when called upon to undertake integrated teaching.
- Students display a high level of anxiety in an integrated curriculum if they are uncertain of the width and depth of a subject they are expected to master.
- The main problem with an integrated curriculum is an attitudinal one, as teachers are protective of their 'territories'.
- While an integrated curriculum may not afford students opportunities to delve deeply into a discipline of interest (except through an elective period of study), students may do so in a topic of interest.

REFERENCES

1 Krathwohl DR. The psychological bases for integration. In: Henry NB, editor. *The Integration of Educational Experiences*, 57th Yearbook of the National Society for the Study of Education, Part III. Chicago, IL: University of Chicago Press; 1958, Chapter III, pp. 43–65.

2 Bloom BS. Ideas, problems and methods of inquiry. In: Henry NB, editor. *The Integration of Educational Experiences*, op. cit., Chapter V, pp. 84–104.

3 Rosse C. Integrated versus discipline-oriented instruction in medical education. *J Med Educ.* 1974; 49: 995–8.

4 Schmidt HG. Problem-based learning: rationale and description. *Med Educ.* 1983; 17: 11–16.

5 McGaghie WC, Miller GE, Sajid AW, *et al.* Competency-based curriculum development in medical education: an introduction. *Public Health Pap.* 1978; 68: 11–91.

6 Lam TP, Irwin M, Chow LW, *et al.* Early introduction of clinical skills teaching in a medical curriculum – factors affecting students' learning. *Med Educ.* 2002; 36: 233–40.

7 Colliver JA. Effectiveness of problem-based learning curricula: research and theory. *Acad Med.* 2000; 75: 259–66.

8 Marton F, Säljö R. On qualitative differences in learning 1. outcome and process, 2. outcome as a function of the learner conception of the task. *Brit J Educ Psychol.* 1976; 46: 4–11, 115–27.

9 Stiernborg M, Bandaranayake R. Medical students' approaches to studying. *Med Teach* 1996; 18: 229–36.

10 Dressel PL. The meaning and significance of integration. In: Henry NB, editor. *The Integration of Educational Experiences*, op. cit., Chapter I, pp. 3–25.

11 Benor DE. Interdisciplinary integration in medical education: theory and method. *Med Educ.* 1982; 16: 355–61.

12 Heylings DJA. Anatomy 1999–2000: the curriculum, who teaches it and how? *Med Educ.* 2002; 36: 702–10.

13 Katz J, Fulop T. Personnel for health care: case studies of educational programmes. *Public Health Pap.* 1978; 70: 1–260.

14 Turnbull EN. Interdisciplinarism: problems and promises. *J Nurs Educ.* 1982; 21: 24–31.

15 Engelberg J. A program of integrative humanistic study for medical students. *Acad Med.* 1992; 67: 455–6.

16 Louw G, Eizenberg N, Carmichael SW. The place of anatomy in medical education: AMEE Guide no 41. *Med Teach.* 2009; 31: 373–86.

17 Jamieson S. Cell and molecular biology in the medical curriculum. *Med Educ.* 2001; 35: 85–6.

18 Collins JP, Gamble GD. A multi-format interdisciplinary final examination. *Med Educ.* 1996; 30: 259–65.

19 Wallace P, Berlin A, Murray E, *et al.* CeMENT: evaluation of a regional development programme integrating hospital and general practice clinical teaching for medical undergraduates. *Med Educ.* 2001; **35**: 160–6.

20 Becher T. The counter-culture of specialisation. *Eur J Educ.* 1990; **25**: 333–46.

21 Mayhew LB. Illustrative courses and programs in colleges and universities. In: Henry NB, editor. *The Integration of Educational Experiences*, op. cit., Chapter XI, pp. 218–48.

22 Bandaranayake RC. A comparison of the reported durations of predominantly integrated and predominantly department-based curricula in North American medical schools (unpublished). Los Angeles, CA: University of Southern California; 1982.

23 Bandaranayake R. The integrated medical curriculum. In: Bandaranayake R, editor. *Trends in Curricula*. Sydney: University of New South Wales Press; 1979. pp. 1–10.

24 Capehart BE. Illustrative courses and programs in selected secondary schools. In: Henry NB, editor. *The Integration of Educational Experiences*, op. cit., Chapter X, pp. 194–217.

25 Prince KJ, van Mameren H, Hylkema N, *et al.* Does problem-based learning lead to deficiencies in basic science knowledge? An empirical case on anatomy. *Med Educ.* 2003; **37**: 15–21.

26 Chrisman LH. Vanishing fences: a parable about educational integration. *J Higher Educ.* 1949; **20**: 242–7.

CHAPTER 6

Integrated student assessment

'Assessment drives learning' is a cliché in medical education, but one that is very accurate. Though one often hears it, the extent to which it is internalised by teachers, and is capitalised on to encourage desirable learning habits in students, is questionable. If integrative learning by students is the aim, how often do we through our assessment systems encourage our students to learn in an integrated manner? Crooks undertook an exhaustive review pertaining to the impact of evaluation on various aspects of student behaviour.[1] He concluded that examinations play a critical role in determining what students learn and how they learn. While many of the studies reviewed determined the effects of assessment practices on learning approaches, retention of information, motivation and critical thinking, studies on the integration of learning were sparse. This chapter will focus on student assessment that is in concordance with the aim of integrated learning.

In Chapter 1 the important role played by assessment in motivating the student to learn in an integrated manner to attain his short-term goals was referred to. Pace pointed out that 'the existence of a need provides direction for behaviour, while the nature of the need determines the extent to which the behaviour is integrative'.[2] An impending examination will encourage students to undertake organised behaviour directed towards satisfying the short-term goals of overcoming that hurdle – that is, to participate in systematic study towards the examination. However, such study will only be integrated if the nature of the examination and the previous learning experiences that preceded self-study were of an integrated nature. The student must be driven to integrated learning by feeling a need for it in order to overcome his short-term goal.

However, in spite of integrated learning experiences, the implicit objectives of a course are evident to students from the nature of its examinations, and these must coincide with students' expectations.[2] If integrated behaviour is seen as accepted and expected behaviour, students develop a mental set for undertaking such behaviour in preparing for examinations. Expectations are determined to a large extent by previous experiences. If the latter have been predominantly of a disciplinary nature, then expectations will also be of that nature and preparation will be geared to satisfying the immediate needs of overcoming the hurdle through undertaking discipline-based study.

An example of this was evident in a medical school that used problem-based learning in one phase of its curriculum. An implicit aim of the school was to produce graduates who were accustomed to undertaking integrated learning so as to adopt an interdisciplinary approach to the solving of clinical and community problems. However, it was commonly observed that the majority of students undertook self-study on a disciplinary basis, even though they were identifying learning needs across the basic medical sciences through interdisciplinary problems. An analysis of the examinations set within and at the end of this phase of the curriculum revealed that many test items were discipline-based, even though they were set within the one question paper or practical examination.[3] It was evident that students' expectations were determined not by the nature of their learning experiences but by that of the examinations to which they and their predecessors were subjected to. They thus undertook discipline-based self-study to satisfy their immediate needs of overcoming the hurdle of the next examination. One aim of the curriculum was thus thwarted. A deliberate attempt was made to increase the degree of integration in the assessment procedures of this school. In a subsequent study on one organ system in this school, students reported that they undertook integrated learning, both between basic and clinical sciences and among the different problems in that system, in reviewing material in preparation for the examination of that organ system.[4] A further study to confirm this finding could focus on the manner in which students answer questions, in such examinations that call upon them to integrate their knowledge.

Planning for learning experiences, their implementation and student assessment are closely related activities.[5] If students are exposed to basic science content in an integrated manner, they should also be assessed in an integrated manner to encourage them to undertake integrated self-study. If the basis for integration is through problems, they should be presented with similar problems in order to assess the extent to which they can demonstrate their integrative capacity. If students are shown how the basic sciences they learn can be applied to clinical and community situations they are likely to encounter in the future (vertical integration), they should be presented with such situations in their examinations to assess their ability to apply basic science knowledge to new situations by interrelating the knowledge they gain from different disciplines. Katz and Fulop state that, even when several courses are taught in parallel, an examination focusing on a specific course may incorporate elements from other courses taught earlier or concomitantly to encourage integrated learning.[6] They also point out the fact that vertical integration is encouraged when the post-test of a given course is based on the prerequisites for a subsequent course.

Many medical schools have replaced subject-based examinations with multi-disciplinary examinations.[7] An assumption is then made that their examinations are thereby integrated. The mere incorporation of test items in a 'multidisciplinary' examination, be it a written paper or a practical station, does not necessarily assess the student's ability to integrate his learning. As emphasised earlier (*see* Chapter 3), the essential ingredient for integration is the establishment of links among the learning from these subjects in relation to a given topic. Thus it is important for a test paper to consist of items, each of which tests these links, rather than of items in each of these subjects.

What types of test items have the potential to test these links?

MULTIPLE-CHOICE QUESTIONS

Multiple-choice questions (MCQ) testing links are difficult but not impossible to construct. Most so-called integrated MCQ, particularly of the multiple-response true–false type (Type X)[8] merely test knowledge from different disciplines in the several response options within the same item. Such items do not really test the student's ability to link one discipline to another. Rather, they test different disciplines separately, similar to a question paper consisting of items from different disciplines. In fact, each response option within a Type X question can be considered a separate test item. If a response option can be constructed in such a way that it tests how the student's knowledge of a given topic in one discipline is related to knowledge of the same topic in another, there is a greater possibility of it being an integrated test item. The more appropriate types of MCQ to test ability to integrate are, however, the single-response type (Type A),[8] or its variation, the extended matching type (Type R),[9] which may test higher cognitive skills of application and problem solving, though not with certainty;[10] and the relationship analysis type (Type E),[8] which requires the student to link an assertion concerning a particular topic to its possible cause. Examples of two of these types, which test links among disciplines, is given here.

Example 1: Single-response (Type A) integrated MCQ

The best evidence for the neuroectodermal origin of the adrenal medulla is that:
1 it has a direct arterial supply from the abdominal aorta
2 its venous drainage is into a persisting part of the subcardinal vein
3 it lies near the sympathetic trunk
4 its secretory cells are innervated by preganglionic fibres
5 its cells show a well-developed granular endoplasmic reticulum.

This item links gross anatomy, embryology, histology and physiology.

Example 2: Relationship-analysis (Type E) integrated MCQ

The ductus arteriosus closes at birth by muscular contraction

because

oxygen tension in the blood perfusing the ductus arteriosus rises when the pulmonary circulation opens up.

This item links embryology and physiology.

FREE-RESPONSE QUESTIONS

Free-response essay questions of various types, such as the long essay, modified essay and short-answer questions, have a greater potential to test integration, even though they are often constructed in a way that they do not call upon the student's ability to display higher-order cognitive skills such as application and problem solving. The knowledge that is often tested by free-response questions can easily be tested more reliably with a series of multiple-choice questions. The great advantage of free-response questions – that is, the ability to test higher cognitive abilities – is lost when they are constructed in this manner. If integration of knowledge is valued, an essay question must focus on testing the student's ability to link knowledge from various disciplines in the same question. The modified essay question has the greatest potential to do so, as it is usually built around a patient or community scenario that is true to life, and proceeds to question the student on various aspects of the chronological development of the initial scenario. Heylings found that all four problem-based curricula that were studied used integrated case-based examinations, while only five of the twelve systems-based curricula, which were not based on problems, used them.[11] There is no reason why an integrated curriculum that is not problem-based should not use problems or cases in its examinations, as they test the student's ability to link knowledge from different disciplines in the solution of the problem, thereby placing the student in real-life practice situations.

Examples of integrated free-response questions are given here.

Example 3: Integrated long essay question

Describe the structural changes associated with the assumption of the erect posture by an infant. List the advantages and disadvantages of each change.

This item tests structure-function relationships.

Example 4: Integrated short-answer question

Name two sites in the body where an intimate relationship between the nervous and endocrine systems is of functional significance. Explain the functional significance of such a relationship at each site, relating function to the histological structure of the site.

This item links histology and physiology.

Example 5: Integrated modified essay question

A modified essay question can be constructed from the following skeleton.

Triggers	Sequence	Questions
Male 25 years admitted to surgical ward	Presents with circumumbilical colicky pain	*Embryology and histology of the appendix*
	Pain is later localised in the right iliac fossa	*Why has the site of the pain changed?*
Abdominal palpation	Tenderness, rigidity and rebound tenderness present	*Innervation of the parietal peritoneum*
Temperature and pulse raised	Complications develop	*Pathogenesis*
Generalised pain	Generalised peritonitis ensues	*Why has the pain changed now?*
Intervention layers	Laparotomy is performed	*Anterior abdominal wall Positions of the appendix*
	Gangrene and perforation occur	*Culture and antibiotics sensitivity*

FIGURE 6.1 Skeleton of an integrated modified essay question

This item links gross anatomy, embryology, histology, neurology, pathology, microbiology and pharmacology.

CLINICAL EXAMINATION

In the clinical examination, the long case has the potential to test the student's ability to integrate the findings from the patient's history, physical examination and investigations in arriving at a differential diagnosis and definitive diagnosis, an advantage that is generally not available in the more focused short case and Objective Structured Clinical Examination (OSCE) or Objective Structured Practical Examination (OSPE). The long case also permits examiners to test the student's knowledge and understanding of underlying basic mechanisms to explain a patient's symptoms and signs in an oral examination.[12] Short cases and OSCEs can test integration among disciplines in a single station if the latter is constructed with due regard to testing links. The use of an 'interdisciplinary'

OSCE involving nine disciplines, to supplement the written papers and long case, was described by Collins and Gamble in the Auckland School of Medicine.[13] However, while this OSCE was multidisciplinary in nature, it did not truly test the students' ability to integrate knowledge from different disciplines as each station focused on a particular discipline. In that sense it was similar to a multi-disciplinary MCQ paper consisting of test items, each of which is unidisciplinary. A truly integrated interdisciplinary OSCE station must test the links among the disciplines within the one station. The feasibility of doing so was stressed by the authors. An example of such a station is given here.

Example 6: An integrated OSCE/OSPE station

Part A. Examine the pathological specimen provided.

1 Name the organ from which this specimen was taken.
2 Describe the macroscopic appearance of the specimen, pointing out particularly its abnormal features.
3 State your diagnostic conclusion from the specimen, justifying your conclusion from the specimen's abnormal features.
4 List the main clinical symptoms and signs you would expect this patient to have shown before his death.

Part B. The histopathological slide provided was taken from a biopsy of the organ.

5 List the histological features seen that either support or do not support your diagnosis.

This station links macroscopic pathology, histopathology and clinical features.

Cox argued that the clinical process is too complex to permit assessment of an integrated clinical performance through structured assessment of its different parts.[14] He advocated judging performance on real-life responsibilities rather than through rigid, contrived situations. Undoubtedly such a strategy would serve integrated assessment well as the assessment is undertaken in the same context in which what is assessed is practised. The logistics of undertaking such a venture in the 'real world' of medical education must be taken into consideration, however valid such a strategy would be for determining clinical competence. Some degree of reality is achieved in the integrated direct observation clinical encounter examination (IDOCEE) devised by Abouna and Hamdy, where the examinee is examined in four stations, each of which is an elongated OSCE involving a patient, and is observed by at least two examiners.[15] Reality is achieved through the duration of each station, which is similar to that which an intern medical officer would spend with a new patient, as well as by the fact that each patient is not identified by speciality or sub-speciality.

AN INSTITUTIONAL SYSTEM FOR CONSTRUCTING INTEGRATED TEST ITEMS

The next issue to consider is the mechanism that a medical school can adopt in order to construct such integrative questions. As long ago as 1958 Mayhew advocated joint meetings among departments to plan examinations that test students' ability to relate material learnt from different courses.[16] When responsibility is given to individual departments to construct questions for an impending examination, teachers tend to adopt an approach that they are comfortable with by confining themselves to their own discipline, and are reluctant to 'tread on the toes' of their colleagues in other departments. In fact some departments object to teachers from other departments encroaching on what they consider their territory when constructing questions. Such an attitude goes against the grain of integration and prevents the ability of a single question to test the links among disciplines. A strategy to overcome this 'territoriality' without detracting from the feeling of power that teachers feel they need to have through examinations was developed in the College of Medicine at the Arabian Gulf University in Bahrain, which was keen to introduce truly integrated questions in its summative examinations. Implementation of the strategy was facilitated by the fact that the curriculum was based on organ-system modules, and the responsibility for both implementation and assessment was in the hands of multidisciplinary committees. The procedure adopted is described here in relation to an integrated modified essay question. However, the same practice can be applied to other types of integrated questions.

About a month before an end-of-module summative examination is due the module committee responsible for that particular organ-system module, or, in the case of an end-of-phase summative examination, the assessment committee responsible for that examination, meets and identifies themes within the module or across modules that are representative of the respective content. An example of a set of themes for the Integumentary System is given in Figure 6.2.[17]

One theme is assigned to each member of the committee, whose responsibility it is to construct questions on the assigned themes. The responsible member constructs the skeleton of a possible question on each theme and discusses it with a subcommittee formed of the relevant disciplines bearing on the proposed question. Each subcommittee member adds 'flesh' to the skeleton, and

Theme	Anatomy	Physiology	Microbiology	Pharmacology	Dermatology
Protective					
Sensory					
Damage					
Immunity					
Infection					

FIGURE 6.2 Themes for an integrated modified essay question on the Integumentary System

the combined effort is discussed at a subsequent meeting of the subcommittee. At this meeting deliberate attempts are made to link the contributions from each discipline in formulating the draft question. The latter is now discussed at a meeting of the module or assessment committee, where further improvements are made before the question is accepted into a bank of questions. The final examination paper is compiled from this bank of questions. The chair of the committee ensures a fair spread across the themes and areas tested in selecting the questions from the bank. In this way, while all relevant departments are involved and sampling issues are addressed, confidentiality is maintained to some degree in setting a truly integrated question paper. Mårtenson *et al.* adopted a similar theme-based integrated final examination in the preclinical phase even when some degree of subject-centred teaching prevailed.[18]

ISSUES IN STUDENT ASSESSMENT IN AN INTEGRATED CURRICULUM

A problem often faced by schools that desire to adopt integrated assessment systems is the manner in which they are required to report scores. In many situations school authorities or higher education bodies require discipline scores, rather than overall scores. Where the unit of integration is, say, an organ system, it is impossible, and in fact undesirable, to report disciplinary scores when questions are truly integrated. This is a good example of a situation in which unnecessary regulations militate against integration. The author is aware of one medical school that had to abandon attempts at curricular integration because of this particular regulation laid down by the accrediting agency appointed by the government. When accrediting bodies are not sufficiently flexible to allow schools to differentiate, but insist on rigid conformity to a particular set of requirements, they inhibit curriculum innovation. There is no real solution to this problem; either the regulation must be withdrawn by the responsible body and the school permitted to report its scores according to the curricular units that form the basis of integration (such as scores in organ systems) or the school must abandon its attempts at integration if it is unwilling to depart from the regulations. As pointed out repeatedly, an integrated curriculum without truly integrated assessment would not lead to integrated learning in the long run.

Another practice that goes against the grain of integration is the credit system that pervades many curricula, particularly North American medical schools and those schools in other countries whose curricula are modelled on this system. Schools that insist on credit allocations to individual disciplines do not promote interdisciplinary integration. The value of such systems in basic medical education, where all students are required to complete the same core courses when training to be non-specialist physicians, is questionable. They are of value only where different courses or curricula need to be equated. The need for equating courses exists where a considerable part of the curriculum is elective in nature;

the need for equating curricula exists when transfer of credits from one school to another is necessitated. Integration should not be sacrificed at the altar of inappropriate systems of quantification of educational experiences. The experience itself, rather than the manner in which it is counted, is of primary importance for the complete education of the budding physician.

National licensing examinations, which are subject-centred, assume a degree of uniformity across schools, and militate against integration and encourage tradition.[19] This was particularly evident in one of the first medical schools to adopt a problem-centred curriculum. On a visit to this school the author became disappointingly aware of the concern that its students displayed about their ability to succeed in an impending national licensing examination that consisted of subject-centred multiple-choice questions. Their concern stemmed from the fact that they lacked confidence in their breadth of knowledge in individual subjects that seemed to be required for successfully passing the examination.

'Harvard reverts to tradition' reported a publication in the journal *Science*.[20] The report referred to an early attempt by the Harvard Medical School to adopt an integrated curriculum,[21] shortly after which it found that there was a significant fall in the average scores of the first class under the new curriculum in the National Board Examination. In their haste to regain their erstwhile pre-eminent position, the school authorities decreed that the curriculum revert to a subject-centred one shortly after the innovation was introduced. What the school, perhaps, failed to realise was that the examination was the culprit rather than the new curriculum; the examination was subject-centred while the curriculum was integrated. National Board examinations were not originally intended to serve the purpose of evaluating the curriculum.[22] It took almost 20 years before Harvard revisited integration in the form of a problem-centred curriculum, fulfilling the predictions of Goldhaber, a second-year medical student in 1973.[20] Western Reserve, which persisted with integration in spite of being placed in the same situation, vis-à-vis the requirement that their students sit the subject-centred national licensing examination, thus became the first medical school to successfully adopt an integrated curriculum. Unless national licensing examinations undergo change, which is congruent with progressive curriculum change, they would not serve the purpose of curriculum improvement.

Another potential threat to integration is the practice of inviting external examiners for the internal examinations of a medical school, ostensibly with the aim of ensuring curriculum standards. In many instances such examiners perform yeoman service in curriculum evaluation with an unbiased perspective. However, if such examiners invited to a school with an integrated curriculum hail from discipline-based schools, they may use evaluative criteria that are more appropriate to their own school rather than the one visited. It is imperative for external examiners to be thoroughly familiar with the nature of the curriculum in the school they visit before they cast judgements on the quality of its education.

Evaluative criteria should be based firmly on the philosophy of the school rather than on personal opinions or preferences.

In the next chapter we will deal with evaluation of the integrated programme, and consider how examinations can be abused in order to show the curriculum 'in good light'. Examinations should be used for the purposes they are intended to serve, one of which is to inculcate good learning habits in students.

KEY POINTS

- Examinations play a critical role in determining what students learn and how they learn.
- Students will prepare for an examination in an integrated manner only if the nature of the examination and the learning experiences that preceded self-study are integrated.
- A multidisciplinary examination is not integrated unless each item within it requires the student to establish links among the disciplines that comprise it.
- An institutional system can be set up that ensures teachers set questions of an integrated nature.
- An administrative requirement to report disciplinary scores goes against the grain of integration, as does the subject credit system practised in many schools.
- A source of great concern to students in an integrated curriculum is the requirement to pass discipline-based national examinations.
- External examiners from schools with discipline-based curricula invited to a school with an integrated curriculum should be familiarised with the nature of the latter before they pass judgements on the quality of its education.

REFERENCES

1 Crooks TJ. The impact of classroom evaluation practices on students. *Rev Educ Res.* 1988; **58**: 438–81.

2 Pace CR. Educational objectives. In: Henry NB, editor. *The Integration of Educational Experiences*, 57th Yearbook of the National Society for the Study of Education, Part III. Chicago, IL: University of Chicago Press; 1958, Chapter IV, pp. 69–83.

3 Al Jafairi ZA. Evaluation of the Integration in Assessment in a Problem-Based Medical School. Unpublished master's thesis, Bahrain: Arabian Gulf University; 2006.

4 Abu-Hijleh MF, Kassab S, Al-Shboul Q, *et al.* Evaluation of the teaching strategy of cardiovascular system in a problem-based curriculum: student perception. *Adv Physiol Educ.* 2004: **28**, 59–63.

5 Capehart BE. Illustrative courses and programs in selected secondary schools. In: Henry NB, editor. *The Integration of Educational Experiences*, op. cit., Chapter X, pp. 194–217.

6 Katz J, Fulop T. Personnel for health care: case studies of educational programmes. *Public Health Pap.* 1978; **70**: 1–260.

7 Benor DE. Interdisciplinary integration in medical education: theory and method. *Med Educ.* 1982; **16**: 355–61.

8 Hubbard JP, Clemans, WV. *Multiple-Choice Examinations in Medicine: a guide for examiner and examinee.* Philadelphia, PA: Lea & Febiger; 1961.

9 Case SM, Swanson DB. Extended matching items: a practical alternative to free-response questions. *Teach Learn Med.* 1993; **5**: 107–15.

10 Cox KR. How did you guess? Or, what do multiple-choice questions measure? *Med J Aust.* 1976; **1**: 384–6.

11 Heylings DJA. Anatomy 1999–2000: the curriculum, who teaches it and how? *Med Educ.* 2002; **36**: 702–10.

12 Foldevi M, Svedin CG. The Linköping curriculum: the phase examination in general practice. *Med Educ.* 1996; **30**: 326–32.

13 Collins JP, Gamble GD. A multi-format interdisciplinary final examination. *Med Educ.* 1996; **30**: 259–65.

14 Cox K. No Oscar for OSCA. *Med Educ.* 1990; **24**: 540–5.

15 Abouna G, Hamdy H. The integrated direct observation clinical encounter examination (IDOCEE) – an objective assessment of students' clinical competence in a problem-based learning curriculum. *Med Teach.* 1999; **21**: 67–72.

16 Mayhew LB. Illustrative courses and programs in colleges and universities. In: Henry NB, editor. *The Integration of Educational Experiences,* op. cit., Chapter XI, pp. 218–48

17 Arabian Gulf University, College of Medicine and Medical Sciences, Phase II Curriculum. Preclinical module examination procedure for Unit VII, Musculoskeletal System. Bahrain: AGU; 1992.

18 Mårtenson D, Håkan A, Kerstin G. An integrated final examination in preclinical subjects for medical students: 10 years of experience. *Teach Learn Med.* 1999; **11**: 26–33.

19 Bandaranayake RC. Implementing change in medical education in developing countries. *Med Teach.* 1989; **11**: 39–45.

20 Goldhaber SZ. Medical education: Harvard reverts to tradition. *Science.* 1973; **181**: 1027–32.

21 Leaf A. Integrating and regrouping courses in the basic medical sciences. In: Lippard VW, Purcell EF, editors. *The Changing Medical Curriculum.* Report of a Macy Conference, New York: Josiah Macy Foundation; 1972, pp. 54–64.

22 Shapiro AP, Schuck RF, Schultz SG, *et al.* The impact of curricular change on performance on National Board examinations. *J Med Educ.* 1974; **49**: 1113–18.

CHAPTER 7

Evaluation of integrated programmes

DEFINITIONS

In this chapter, programme evaluation, as distinct from student assessment, will be considered in relation to either the establishment of new integrated programmes or the replacement of an existing discipline-based programme with a more integrated one.

Programme evaluation is a process of obtaining and using information about the various components of a programme as a basis for making decisions pertaining to that programme.[1] It differs from conclusion-oriented research, which is directed towards generating new knowledge.[2] The term 'evaluation' implies a value judgement. Such judgement is based on certain measurements or assessments made about various components of the programme. This judgement is made against implicit or explicit standards. All judgement involves a degree of subjectivity, but it is the evaluator's duty to be as objective as possible.

THE FOCUS OF EVALUATION

Student assessment, which was considered in Chapter 6, specifically involves obtaining data from various sources about the abilities of the student. Based on these data certain value judgements are made about the student's abilities, against standards that are either norm-referenced or criterion-referenced. Since, as pointed out in Chapter 1, the curriculum is a system of interrelated components, and the students are one of these components, student assessment data may contribute to programme evaluation. However, as will be shown, caution must be exercised in using student assessment data to make value judgements about a curriculum.

While many aspects of an integrated curriculum may be evaluated, in this chapter the focus is specifically the degree and effects of integration undertaken by both students, in their learning, and teachers, in the extent to which they facilitate such learning. Integration may be evident in both the plan and the process of a curriculum. However, while the curriculum plan may indicate considerable potential for integrated learning by students, the actual implementation of the plan may not. This is because the 'curriculum on paper' may not correspond with the 'curriculum in practice', as discussed in Chapter 1. Thus while the curriculum plan is one component of curriculum evaluation, it is inadequate to base one's judgements on the plan alone; data pertaining to the degree of integration in the curriculum processes must also be obtained. In addition, even if the processes implemented in the curriculum may show integrative activity by both students and faculty, what ultimately matters is the extent to which students show integrative capacity in the way in which they *use* their learning. The extent to which students are able to link what they learn from different courses, disciplines, modalities of learning and loci of learning, and then form meaningful 'wholes' that demonstrate their ability to apply such learning when faced with novel situations, is indicative of the degree of successful integrative learning they have undertaken. Such learning in students is a product (or output) of the curriculum. This leads us to one of the models of curriculum evaluation; namely, the 'context-input-process-product' (CIPP) model for decision-oriented evaluation proposed by Stufflebeam *et al.*[3]

A PROGRAMME EVALUATION MODEL

Of all the models available for evaluating an integrated programme, Stufflebeam's CIPP model seems to be most apt. This model closely resembles Donabedian's structure-process-outcomes paradigm in the field of health quality assurance.[4] Stufflebeam's model for programme evaluation will be illustrated in relation to an integrated programme (*see* Figure 7.1).

Each of the components in Figure 7.1 can be the focus of evaluation. These components are considered in the four categories of context, input, process and product. They are only given as examples; undoubtedly, evaluators may wish to consider other components that may be of particular interest to them in a given situation.

If we take each of these categories in turn we can see how we can relate evaluation questions to the specific characteristics of an integrated curriculum.

INPUT	PROCESS	PRODUCT
students	learning	graduate abilities
teachers	teaching	teacher satisfaction
curriculum plan	assessment	interdepartmental harmony
facilities	committee meetings	institutional recognition
administration	decision-making	institutional role model

CONTEXT: tradition; requirements by higher authorities; accreditation

FIGURE 7.1 The CIPP model of programme evaluation[3] applied to a curriculum

Context

This forms the milieu in which the school functions and has an important bearing on the school's ability to undertake curriculum integration.

➤ Tradition:
  — To what extent does the tradition of the academic society in which the medical school is situated militate against an integrated curriculum?
  — Does the school have close ties with an older, traditional school that interferes with its ability to implement an integrated curriculum?

➤ Requirements by higher authorities:
  — Is there a requirement by a higher authority, such as the Ministry of Higher Education, that the school conforms to a given set of guidelines that interferes with the implementation of an integrated curriculum?
  — Do licensing requirements, such as by a national board, insist on candidates demonstrating proficiency in individual disciplines?
  — Does a rigid credit system, which insists on stipulated hours and/or sequence of training in individual disciplines, prevail in the school?

➤ Accreditation:
  — To what extent does the system of institutional accreditation encourage curriculum integration?
  — Do members of the accrediting team have disciplinary biases?
  — What proportion of the members of the accreditation team come from schools with an integrated curriculum?

Inputs

These are the elements that are *prerequisite* to curriculum implementation.

➤ Students:
  — What proportion of medical students admitted to the school comes from a traditional high school background that fosters didactic methods of instruction?
  — What are the proportions of medical students who favour surface and deep learning among those who enter the integrated curriculum?
  — What proportion of medical students admitted has difficulties in the medium of instruction that prevent them from benefitting from, or contributing to, those parts of the curriculum that are integrated?

➤ Teachers:
  — How many teachers have experienced an integrated curriculum previously?
  — Are teachers willing to communicate and collaborate with their colleagues in other departments?
  — Are there any serious antagonists to the concept of curriculum integration among the teachers in the school and how influential are they?

➤ Curriculum plan:
  — Do the general objectives in the curriculum plan emphasise the need to relate learning from different components of the curriculum?
  — Does the curriculum plan afford opportunities for students to learn different subjects simultaneously?
  — Does the curriculum plan foster (a) self-directed learning; (b) application of previous learning; (c) reinforcement of previous learning; (d) problem solving; (e) relating learning to living?
  — Does the curriculum plan promote assessments where previous learning can be assessed in subsequent examinations?
➤ Facilities:
  — What proportions of (a) textbooks and (b) reference books in the school's library deal with the disciplines in an integrated manner?
  — Are the textbooks prescribed for students strictly unidisciplinary?
  — Are there audio-visual resources that deal with topics in an integrated manner available to students for self-study?
  — How many laboratories in the school are multidisciplinary in nature?
➤ Administration:
  — Does the Head of the institution (e.g. dean) support an integrated curriculum?
  — Are budget allocations for teaching purposes made on a departmental basis?

Processes

These are the activities undertaken during implementation of the curriculum.
➤ Student learning:
  — When students undertake self-study, do they attempt to link their learning from different (a) disciplines, (b) units, (c) phases of the curriculum?
  — During problem-based learning tutorials, do students demonstrate the need and willingness to link content from different (a) disciplines, (b) problems, (c) units?
  — Do student learn to apply learning from previous (a) problems, (b) units, (c) phases of the curriculum when studying at a later stage?
  — What proportion of students preparing for an examination does so in an integrated way, rather than according to disciplines?
  — Do students practise application of concepts and principles to problems during their learning?
➤ Teaching:
  — To what extent do individual teachers show links among disciplines and units when implementing their teaching activities?
  — Do teachers, including service providers who function as part-time

teachers, act as good role models to students in their daily interactions with (a) patients, (b) community, (c) other members of the healthcare team?
— To what extent do team members teaching students simultaneously complement each other?
— Do teachers demonstrate the link between theoretical and practical components of a unit?
— Do teachers show the relevance of what they teach to the students' future roles?
➤ Assessment:
— Are summative examinations planned by interdisciplinary or departmental groups?
— What proportion of test items in the individual components of an examination calls upon the students' ability to link their learning from different (a) disciplines (b) units (c) phases of the curriculum?
— To what extent are clinical teachers involved in basic science examinations, and vice versa?
— How close to reality are the conditions under which students are examined in the final qualifying examination?
➤ Committee meetings:
— Is curriculum planning undertaken by interdisciplinary committees?
— Do teachers in a given unit collaborate in planning the specific teaching activities of that unit before it is implemented?
— How often does the committee for overseeing the implementation and planning of the whole curriculum meet?
— Does the committee for evaluating the curriculum pay particular attention to determining whether the objectives related to integration are met?

Products
These are the consequences of implementing the curriculum.
➤ Graduates:
— To what extent are the graduates of the school able to recall basic principles they learnt in the curriculum and apply them to practice?
— To what extent are the graduates adept at solving problems that they confront in practice?
— To what extent are graduates of the school sought after by clinical supervisors?
➤ Teachers:
— What is the degree of satisfaction expressed by teachers about the curriculum?
— To what extent do teachers say that they have gained in learning by participating in an integrated curriculum?

— To what extent is there interdisciplinary harmony among teachers from different disciplines on matters pertaining to the curriculum?
➤ Institutional recognition:
  — How recognised is the school at a (a) national (b) international level?
  — Has the school served as an 'institutional role model' to other schools planning or implementing integrated curricula?
  — Has the school been the recipient of any awards because of the nature of its curriculum?
  — Has the school received accolades from visiting groups, such as accreditation teams, because of its curriculum?

These are some examples of evaluation questions that may be asked in order to evaluate an integrated curriculum. It is not an exhaustive list; in fact no list can be exhaustive, as there are a myriad of foci for investigating a curriculum. Each of these questions subsumes many other questions before the evaluator can get to the stage where the evaluation question is specific enough to obtain data to answer it. The mushrooming nature of evaluation questions as they become increasingly specific, and operational, precludes dealing with too many of them. Thus it is necessary for the evaluator to determine priorities for evaluation.

PRIORITIES FOR EVALUATION

There are many techniques for determining priorities for evaluation, and all of them involve some degree of subjectivity. A common technique is the nominal group process or a modified version of it.[5] The most important factor to take into consideration in determining priorities for evaluation is the degree of concern that the stakeholders of the programme indicate. Concerns arise from perceived deficiencies in the programme. The 'deficiency model' of evaluation focuses on perceived deficiencies and goes on to confirm the deficiency and identify the factors responsible for its existence. Thus if a perceived deficiency is, say, that students in the integrated curriculum undertake rote learning in spite of its integrated nature, the evaluator first confirms that this is in fact true to the extent that it is a cause for concern, and then tries to delineate the reasons for this deficiency. In delineating the possible reasons for its existence, many evaluation questions must be asked and each investigated. A single question may thus mushroom into several, making it difficult for the evaluator to investigate more than a few questions.

Another important factor to take into consideration in determining priorities is the potential of the focus of evaluation for programme improvement. It is obvious that the primary purpose of evaluating a programme is to enable decisions to be made in order to either improve it or abandon it. Improvement of a programme can occur in two ways: by capitalising on its strengths or reducing its deficiencies. Logically, there is more room for improvement by reducing deficiencies than by capitalising on strengths. Thus the deficiency model of evaluation is of particular significance for programme improvement. Some educators, however, take exception to a negativistic approach to evaluation engendered by this model, and bemoan the fact that the strengths of the programme are not highlighted by this approach. This is a genuine concern, and should be addressed by not confining evaluation to questions related to deficiencies.

When an existing curriculum, or part of it, is replaced by an integrated one, the focus of evaluation should relate to the purposes of the change. The trigger for the change may have been some perceived or established concerns or deficiencies in the curriculum, and the new programme instituted to correct those deficiencies. In the early years of the change, evaluation should focus on those deficiencies, and information obtained to determine whether they are being corrected by the new curriculum. In later years, programme evaluation can be undertaken to determine if the intended changes are being maintained. Problem-based learning, for example, has been introduced in many medical curricula because it is supposed to encourage a deep learning approach in students, requiring them to understand and integrate the learning from different disciplines that are relevant to the problem at hand. A study undertaken by Dolmans *et al.* at the University of Limburg Medical School in Maastricht, long after this method of learning was introduced in the school, showed that 'PBL [problem-based learning] students seem to use a deep approach rather than a surface approach, although the second year students tend to have a somewhat less deep approach and more surface approach than first year students'.[6] They hypothesised that this difference could possibly be due to the former's perception that they need not study in depth to obtain a sufficient mark on the test in Year 2. If this is so, faculty should be guided to improve their assessment procedures in Year 2 in order to encourage deep learning.

The replacement of a conventional curriculum with an integrated one offers an excellent opportunity to compare the old and new curricula, as the former is being phased out while the latter is being introduced. The author had such an opportunity as chairman of a course evaluation committee when a new curriculum was being introduced at the University of New South Wales in Sydney.[7] Using the same data-collecting instruments, each year of the old curriculum was evaluated simultaneously with the corresponding year of the new curriculum using a variety of methods. A limitation of this comparison was that, necessarily, cohorts of students pursuing courses in a given year of the curriculum were compared at different times, rather than at the same time, as would have been possible if parallel tracks of the old and new curricula were implemented simultaneously. In spite of this limitation the evaluators were able to provide evidence as to whether the goals of the curriculum change were being met in the new curriculum better than in the old.

A comparison of students in parallel tracks was undertaken in the medical school in Michigan State University, as pointed out in Chapter 4 (personal communication, 1982). One track was subject-centred, like most American medical schools at the time, with the exception that a few focal problems were introduced in each course to develop students' skills in problem solving and their ability to apply basic sciences in so doing. The second track, which was problem-based, commenced on an experimental basis in 1974 and was established more firmly in 1978. While the outcomes in cognitive performance between the two groups were found to be comparable, the second group of graduates was found to be more confident, more socially interactive, more committed to self-directed learning and to embark more often on primary care careers. It was perhaps tempting for the proponents of the second track to conclude that these differences were the result of the different training this group was subjected to. To their credit, however, they concluded that the differences may have arisen from the fact that, at admission, students were asked to volunteer for either track, and that the more mature students opted for the second track. Colliver identified pre-existing differences between non-randomised groups as one of the problems confronting the evaluator attempting to compare problem-based and standard curricula.[8] Comparative studies should account for possible confounding variables before one type of curriculum can be judged superior to another. The difficulty in controlling confounding variables in studies is one reason for the lack of clear evidence in the literature of the superiority of integrated (including problem-centred) curricula over conventional ones.

Another difficulty in comparison is the use of inappropriate yardsticks, biased towards one type of curriculum, for comparison. Scores on discipline-based national board examinations, for example, are inappropriate to evaluate an integrated curriculum. The earlier experience of Harvard Medical School with an integrated curriculum was referred to in Chapter 6. The ranking of schools on performance in such examinations cannot be used to determine the relative merits of curricula.

THE USES OF PROGRAMME EVALUATION

This brings us to the uses of programme evaluation. As with all evaluation exercises the question: 'How are the results of evaluation to be used?' must be asked. In the initial stages of implementing an integrated curriculum, monitoring of the new curriculum must be maintained from the outset. 'Teething difficulties' are bound to occur, and they must be identified and dealt with. This means that programme evaluation must be planned after the curriculum is planned but before its implementation commences. Perceptions of stakeholders must be sought early for these difficulties to be identified. In the University of New South Wales study referred to previously[7] we sought these perceptions from students and teachers midway through each course, when it was first implemented in the new curriculum. This timing gave both groups enough time to identify difficulties, as well as to make any mid-course corrections if necessary. O'Hanlon et al. sought the perceptions of first-year medical students to a problem-based learning module in behavioural sciences introduced for the first time.[9] Students perceived the module to be interesting but less beneficial than the traditional approach. More important, they perceived the need for more guidance on what was expected of them, as well as for background information on the topic before the tutorials. Such perceptions could provide guidance to the teachers on ways of improving the module without compromising the philosophy of problem-based learning.

Faculty perceptions are as important, not only from the point of view of correcting course deficiencies, but also to maintain faculty morale and attitudes to teaching. Finucane *et al.* compared teachers at a traditional and an innovative school, and found that they perceived both intrinsic rewards (internal satisfaction) and extrinsic rewards (recognition and promotion) to be greater in the innovative school.[10] Early detection of faculty attitudes to a newly introduced integrated curriculum is important for either capitalising on positive attitudes or arriving at compromises if negative attitudes predominate.

A common practice in programme evaluation is to determine respondents' satisfaction levels in relation to specific aspects of the programme.[11] Satisfaction levels are, of course, subjective, and do not necessarily give 'hard' data on which decisions can be based. They are important, nevertheless, as they may give pointers as to which aspects of the programme need to be investigated further.

Summative evaluation must be undertaken when each course in the new curriculum is completed. The purpose of such evaluation is to provide data to committees responsible for course management and implementation to make decisions pertaining to changes to each year of the new curriculum before it is re-implemented the following year. Summative evaluation is usually focused on the products of the programme, but may include elements of the process that are of particular concern. One of the products in summative evaluation is student performance. Results of student assessment must be treated with caution when used as an indicator to evaluate programmes. The author is acutely aware of some faculty members who are so apprehensive of high failure rates that particular care is taken to prevent such through devious undesirable practices, in order to show the curriculum in good light. Suchman has labelled such biased evaluation as 'whitewash'.[12]

The ultimate goal of medical education is to produce physicians who would provide quality healthcare. Thus the most important standards of programme evaluation are those that are related to the quality of care. Long-term evaluation of the products of a particular curriculum is undertaken with this in mind. One indicator for long-term evaluation that has been used is the ratings obtained from the supervisors of the graduates of the programme. The evaluator has to be cautious about the possible presence of the 'halo effect' in evaluations undertaken by some supervisors, who may only identify gross deficiencies. Nevertheless, supervisor ratings may give valuable evidence of the short-term outcomes of the products of the curriculum. An indirect indicator of supervisor preferences is the proportion of graduates from a given school who are successful in obtaining their first priority for internship or residency training, in those countries where graduates have the opportunity to apply for training positions. If over a period of time graduates from a particular school obtain a significantly larger proportion of first priorities compared with those from another school or from all schools, this is an unobtrusive measure of supervisor preferences for the graduates of the former school. Another unobtrusive measure is the extent to which the innovation is accepted by other schools in the region, or other faculties within the university.

Any major curriculum development must have an in-built plan for long-term evaluation of its output. Outcome measures are fraught with the danger of contamination by extraneous variables not directly related to the curriculum. They tend to even out over time, irrespective of the school of which the graduate is a product. Herein is one difficulty in comparing, say, an integrated curriculum with a conventional one. Nevertheless, such methods as career-tracking, graduate follow-up and postgraduate performance give important measures of the quality of the product.

Some of these studies may be of a qualitative nature. The earliest school to introduce an integrated curriculum, Western Reserve Medical School, had the foresight to plan a comparative study of six batches of its graduates from the old and the new curricula, through visits to their practice locations two and five years after graduation (personal communication, 1973). One particular finding of interest was that graduates of the old curriculum tended to remember good and poor *teachers*, while those of the new curriculum remembered good and poor *courses*.

THE EVALUATOR

An important question to ask is: 'Who should evaluate?' Evaluation can be undertaken by both 'insiders' (i.e. those who are part of the institution and take an active part in the programme being evaluated) or 'outsiders' (i.e. those who have no stake in the programme being evaluated). Accrediting teams, for example, play the role of external evaluators. Each of these categories has its advantages and disadvantages. The internal evaluator is intimately associated with the programme and is most likely to know its aims and nature. However, she is also more likely to be biased in the evaluation, because the outcomes of evaluation may affect her directly. On the other hand, if the internal evaluator undertakes an honest evaluation of the programme, utilisation of the results of evaluation is more likely to take place, because of the sense of ownership that the school has of the evaluation.

The external evaluator is less likely to be affected by biases, and more likely to paint a truer picture of the value of the programme. However, when external evaluators from a discipline-based medical school are invited to undertake an evaluation of an integrated curriculum, or a course within it, they may tend to use standards that are not appropriate to the integrated curriculum. As pointed out in Chapter 6, external evaluators need to be thoroughly familiarised with the philosophy of the curriculum, its sequence and the objectives of the courses they evaluate before they pass comparative judgements on either the calibre of the students or the value of the courses. As Moy pointed out, 'the unusual academic structure . . . is often of concern to faculty members from traditional schools who find themselves visiting new schools as part of accreditation survey teams'.[13]

The concerned evaluator has to tread a tightrope between insider and outsider status, capitalising on being an outsider, yet viewing the implementation of the curriculum from the inside, without being subjected to the biases if an insider. He often has to arrive at a compromise of

> negotiated purpose and process, where [he]: declares purpose and procedure, but is willing to negotiate; increases client participation in policy and process to enhance utilization of results; recognizes the client's right to know what he is doing and why; and ensures that all clients have some stake in the evaluation process.[14]

The evaluator's role is not an easy one. He is often a lonely figure in a stormy world, buffetted by administrative, academic and political forces, trying to juggle several balls at the same time and keep them all going, often subjected to brickbats, rarely bouquets, yet crucial to the success of the programme. Knowledge, skills and, above all, attitudes are his enduring weapons.

KEY POINTS

- The curriculum plan is inadequate to base one's judgement on the degree of integration; data pertaining to the process of integration must also be obtained.
- In an integrated curriculum, the product of learning of specific interest is the extent to which students are able to link what they learn from different segments of the curriculum.
- The mushrooming nature of evaluation questions as they become increasingly specific necessitates limiting evaluation to priority concerns pertaining to the curriculum.
- If the purpose of evaluation is programme improvement, there is more room for improvement by correcting deficiencies than by capitalising on strengths.
- The replacement of a conventional curriculum by an integrated one offers an excellent opportunity to compare the old and new curricula.
- Comparative studies should account for potential confounding variables before one type of curriculum can be judged superior to another.

- Programme evaluation must be planned after curriculum planning but before its implementation.
- Student and faculty perceptions during implementation are important for monitoring a new curriculum so that mid-course corrections can be made.
- Summative evaluation at the end of the course should provide data for decision-makers on indicated changes for succeeding years.
- The most important standards of evaluation of a curriculum are those related to the quality of care provided by its products.
- The evaluator has to tread a tightrope between 'insider' and 'outsider' status, becoming thoroughly familiar with the programme being evaluated, while avoiding the biases of stakeholders.

REFERENCES

1 Coles CR, Grant JG. Curriculum evaluation in medical and health-care education. *Med Educ.* 1985; **19**: 405–42.

2 Rotem A, Bandaranayake R. How to plan and conduct programme evaluation. *Med Teach.* 1983; **5**: 127–31.

3 Stufflebeam DL, Foley WJ, Gephart WJ, *et al. Educational Evaluation and Decision Making.* Itasca, IL: Peacock; 1971.

4 Donabedian A. Quality assessment and monitoring: retrospect and prospect. *Eval Health Prof.* 1983; **6**: 363–75.

5 Delbecq AL, VandeVen AH. A group process model for problem identification and program planning. *J Appl Behav Sci.* 1971; **7**: 466–91.

6 Dolmans DH, Wolfhagen IH, Ginns P. Measuring approaches to learning in a problem based learning context. *Int J Med Educ.* 2010; **1**: 55–60.

7 Craig P, Bandaranayake R. Experiences with a method for obtaining feedback on a medical curriculum undergoing change. *Med Educ.* 1993; **27**: 15–21.

8 Colliver JA. Effectiveness of PBL curricula (Letters to the Editor). *Med Educ.* 2000; **34**: 959–60.

9 O'Hanlon A, Winefield H, Hejka E, *et al.* Initial responses of first-year medical students to problem-based learning in a behavioural science course: role of language background and course content. *Med Educ.* 1995; **29**: 198–204.

10 Finucane P, Allery LA, Hayes TM. Comparison of teachers at a 'traditional' and an 'innovative' medical school. *Med Educ.* 1995; **29**: 104–9.

11 Antepohl W, Domeij E, Forsberg P, *et al.* A follow-up of medical graduates of a problem-based learning curriculum. *Med Educ.* 2003; **37**: 155–62.

12 Suchman EA. *Evaluation Research,* New York, NY: Russell Sage Foundation; 1967.

13 Moy RH. Critical values in medical education. *N Engl J Med.* 1979; **301**: 694–7.

14 Eraut M. Handling value issues. In: Adelman C, editor. *The Politics and Ethics of Evaluation.* London: Croom-Helm; 1984, pp. 26–42.

CHAPTER 8

Pitfalls and guidelines

This chapter draws upon some of the principles and practices presented in the previous chapters to:

1 highlight the common pitfalls that an established traditional medical school desirous of changing to an integrated curriculum, or a new school intending to institute one, is likely to encounter

2 provide some guidelines that may be followed to optimise the chances of such a curriculum being successful.

PITFALLS IN IMPLEMENTATION

A clear understanding of the concept of integration by all participants in the planning and implementation stages is critical if any attempt to introduce an integrated curriculum is to succeed. In an unreported study conducted several years ago in one medical school that had decided to change from a subject-centred to an integrated curriculum, individual interviews were conducted with teachers in several departments of the school to determine their perception of the concept of integration. It came as no surprise that there were many interpretations of the concept. Some perceived integration as adding different components together ('summation'); some as arranging curriculum components in a logical order ('sequencing'); some as teaching related parts, for example structure and function of an organ, together ('synchronisation'); some as teaching undertaken by teachers in different disciplines together ('team teaching'). Rarely did faculty perceive integration as linking content from different disciplines. In a recent study, Muller *et al.* found similar differences among stakeholder groups in their interpretation of an integrated curriculum.[1] Clearly such different interpretations thwart useful discussion in the planning stage of the innovation, and may lead to different practices in the implementation stage. Katz and Fulop pointed out that varying interpretation of the concept 'could lead to conflicts even among well-meaning and motivated colleagues', not only among those who disagree with the philosophy.[2]

A second critical factor is determining and agreeing on a common set of goals and general objectives for the curriculum. As long ago as 1954, Dupont stated that one of the greatest weaknesses of curricular plans is the lack of a common philosophy between curriculum planners and implementers.[3] In a study involving five North American medical schools that taught medical students an integrated approach to healthcare, addressing 'the complex interaction of many factors influencing health and illness', Tresolini *et al.* found that a 'strongly held, broadly shared mission or philosophy in focusing attention on both biomedical and non-biomedical concerns' was most important.[4] If there is disagreement on the nature of the end product that the school wishes to train, then integration would surely fail. Agreement is enhanced by communication among departments, among different levels within departments and throughout the institution, an activity that is generally minimal in the busy lives of medical school faculty.[2] When implementers are not consulted during the planning stages of any innovation, the likelihood of successful implementation of the plan is minimal. This is because of a lack of ownership of the plan by the implementers.

As with any innovation, traditionalism is a common deterrent to integration. Universities are notoriously slow in introducing change, as change implies deviation from what has been established and carries the potential risk of non-acceptance by teachers, students and society. Teachers are comfortable with what they are accustomed to, students are apprehensive of the effects of the change on their learning and examination performance, administrators are concerned about the costs associated with the change and society is wary of the effects of the change on standards of practice. Traditionalism is often supported by nebulous educational standards, which frustrate introduction and maintenance of relevant education.[2] Accrediting and professional bodies have, in the past, often exerted pressure on schools to maintain and improve traditional curricula rather than bring about major change that would overhaul the system.[3] However, a current trend among accrediting bodies is to encourage change and judge each school against its philosophy, as long as the ultimate goals of medical education are achieved. This principle is clearly enunciated in the guidelines laid down by the Australian Medical Council for Australian and New Zealand medical schools preparing for accreditation.[5]

Discipline-based departments are useful for research and tertiary patient care but are a major barrier to attempts at introducing an integrated curriculum. Teachers are trained and gain postgraduate experience in specific disciplines and sub-disciplines. In the basic science departments such postgraduate training is often research-based. Following an intensive period of immersion in a narrow area of training and specialisation, it is natural for teachers, particularly in the period immediately following postgraduate training, to focus all their efforts, including teaching and research, on this narrow area. Reluctance to participate in teaching in an integrated curriculum, where many disciplines combine within the same teaching session, is exacerbated by their lack of familiarity with areas beyond their purview. Thus particular care must be taken when involving junior teachers in implementing an integrated curriculum. For successful implementation it is important to have on board teachers who have themselves integrated their knowledge.[6] This is unlikely to be the case with recently specialised teachers who have either just joined an institution or just returned after postgraduate training. On the other hand, reluctance of senior teachers to participate in integrated teaching is often attitudinal and stems from the reluctance to deviate from their 'comfort zone'. Thus a strategy of involvement needs to be adopted in convincing them of the value of the change.

Teachers who are accustomed to regarding curricula as consisting of subjects, rather than as a system with interrelated components, fail to realise that change in one component of the system warrants appropriate changes in other components. The effect of incongruent examinations was pointed out in Chapter 6. The same is true when courses consist of interdisciplinary content but learning experiences are organised in a manner that leaves each department to make its contribution independently of the other departments. Special attention must be paid to interdepartmental organisation[7] and sequencing of integrated learning experiences.[2] Many of these points have been taken into consideration by Rotem and Bandaranayake[8] in developing a framework for analysis to improve medical education.

GUIDELINES FOR IMPLEMENTATION

1 A clear *understanding* of the concept of integration, and of the need to link contributions from different disciplines to achieve wholeness in what the student learns, must be attained by all planners and implementers of the curriculum if it is to promote real integrated learning. Faculty development activities that focus on this key characteristic, replete with examples highlighting links among the various disciplines, must be conducted from the outset of the curriculum-planning exercise.

2 Once understanding of the concept has been attained, *acceptance* of the philosophy should be sought. There are bound to be antagonists to the philosophy, often with genuine reasons for concern. Attempts should be made to win them over through meetings where they are free to express their concerns and discuss them without fear of repercussion. In spite of this, if a large proportion of the faculty still doubt the value of the philosophy, a curricular experiment should be set up on a small segment of the curriculum that is carefully planned, implemented and evaluated. If there is general resistance by disciplinary experts to give away courses previously taught on a unidisciplinary basis for such an experiment, a new integrated course should be selected on a topic, such as nutrition or medical ethics, which would lend itself to the experiment. Anxiety among the doubters may often be allayed through direct experience in the process of integration. The seeking of teacher and student opinion about the experience immediately after it is completed

may help to dispel these fears and doubts. Enforcing a practice on an unwilling faculty, through administrative fiat or regulation, should be avoided at all cost, as the change would surely fail in the long run. The presence of a growing critical mass of teachers in favour of the change would augur well for its success.

3 While it is impossible for all teachers to take part in planning exercises, these exercises should not be the sole domain of a select few; as many as possible should be involved through the establishment of committees and subcommittees for various phases and modules of the curriculum. Those who are not directly involved in planning, but who are likely to be the future implementers of the plan, should be kept constantly informed of the stages of development of the plan, and their opinions sought and views addressed at each stage. Planning committees should be genuinely representative of the relevant departments and disciplines when a particular part of the curriculum is being planned. Special attention should be given to interdisciplinary planning and organisation of the curriculum. Where vertical integration is valued, planning committees should incorporate clinical and community medicine teachers as appropriate.

4 When the curriculum framework has been agreed upon, planning of the details of each organisational unit should be entrusted to an interdisciplinary committee consisting of disciplinary representatives most appropriate for the unit. Such committees should be selected carefully as it is likely, and desirable, that they will also be responsible for the implementation of their respective units after the curriculum has been planned. This follows the principle that participation in planning increases ownership, which facilitates successful implementation. Most important, each unit should not be seen as the responsibility of a given department but of the interdisciplinary committee to which it was assigned. Departmental input should be through the respective representative, who should truly represent the respective department's opinion rather than his own. Any attempt by a given department to take over the implementation of a planned unit should be resisted at all cost. The role of departmental Heads as far as the curriculum is concerned is ensuring that both human and physical resources within the department are made available for curriculum implementation. Each department should form a departmental committee, chaired by the Head, to discuss its input into the integrated curriculum, and how best it can contribute to the philosophy of integration. Nevertheless, the ultimate authority as far as a given unit is concerned is the unit committee. Specific goal statements, to which agreement is obtained, are critically important for coordinating a course involving large numbers of instructors.[9]

5 Teaching activities that facilitate integrated learning should be planned. The tendency to revert to accustomed methods of teaching should be curbed.

Whenever possible, problem-based learning, problem-solving exercises, team-based learning,[10] case-based learning, clinically-oriented seminars and clinicopathological conferences should be substituted for lectures. The latter should be confined to topics that students have difficulty understanding or accessing suitable reading material on. Similarly, multidisciplinary laboratories, integrated practical classes and clinical skill laboratories in which both basic science and clinical teachers participate should be substituted for unidisciplinary practical classes, whenever possible.

6 Particular attention should be paid to planning integrated assessment instruments. Many teachers are unaware of the nature of integrated test items and need to be trained. The strategy outlined in Chapter 6 could be followed in developing integrated examinations. The unit committee should have responsibility for the assessment of students in each unit, while an examinations committee consisting of the chairs of all units in a given phase should have responsibility for summative assessment of the phase. Both basic science and clinical summative assessments should incorporate items that test application of the basic sciences to clinical and community health situations, in order to encourage vertical integration.

7 Faculty training is critical if the integrated curriculum is to be successfully established and maintained. Teachers are usually not accustomed to this curriculum model, and are thus apprehensive of teaching in such a curriculum. Training includes developing integrated lesson plans, conducting joint teaching sessions and constructing integrated test items and stations.

8 A plan for curriculum evaluation should be developed before the integrated curriculum is implemented. This plan should, if the integrated curriculum is replacing a subject-centred one, be such that a comparison between the two is made possible during each phase. The main objective of evaluation is to determine whether the primary purpose of the change – that is, to encourage students to undertake integrated learning – is being met. Formative course evaluation should be such that deficiencies could be identified on an ongoing basis so that mid-course corrections could be made. Careful determination of the reasons for the existence of 'teething problems' during the early stages of implementation would prevent hurried or drastic measures being taken inappropriately. Detailed reporting and discussion of evaluation reports with relevant committees would encourage protagonists and allay the fears of antagonists. Compromises may have to be made, and planners must be careful not to be too rigid in their opinions when evaluation results indicate modification or adaptation. Most important, willingness to keep an open mind about any curriculum change would prevent the innovation of today becoming the tradition of tomorrow.

KEY POINTS

- A clear understanding of the concept of integration by planners and implementers is critical.
- A common set of goals and general objectives must be determined and agreed upon.
- Traditionalism is a common deterrent to integration.
- As many implementers as possible should be involved in planning to create a sense of ownership and commitment to the plan.
- Interdepartmental committees should be responsible for managing segments of the curriculum, with relevant departments being truly represented in each committee.
- The tendency to revert to accustomed methods of teaching, contrary to the philosophy of integration, should be curbed.
- Particular attention should be paid to truly integrated test items in student assessment procedures.
- Faculty training is essential for successful implementation.
- A programme evaluation plan should be developed before implementation commences.

REFERENCES

1 Muller JH, Jain S, Loeser H, *et al.* Lessons learned about integrating a medical school curriculum: perceptions of students, faculty and curriculum leaders. *Med Educ.* 2008; **42**: 778–85.

2 Katz J, Fulop T. Personnel for health care: case studies of educational programmes. *Public Health Pap.* 1978; **70**: 1–260.

3 Dupont GE. Toward an integrated curriculum. *J Amer Assoc Collegiate Registrars* 1954; **29**: 197–214.

4 Tresolini CP, Shugars DA, Lee LS. Teaching an integrated approach to health care: lessons from five schools. *Acad Med.* 1995; **70**: 665–70.

5 Australian Medical Council. *The Assessment and Accreditation of Medical Schools by the Australian Medical Council.* Canberra: Australian Medical Council; 1992.

6 Knudson CW. What do educators mean by integration? *Harv Educ Rev.* 1937; **7**: 15–26.

7 Davis WK, White B-A. Centralized decision making in management of the curriculum at the University of Michigan Medical School. *Acad Med.* 1993; **68**: 333–5.

8 Rotem A, Bandaranayake R. Difficulties in improving medical education: a framework for analysis. *Higher Education.* 1981; **10**: 597–603.

9 Talalla A, Boufford JI, Lass SL. An integrated clinical correlation course in the neurosciences for first-year medical students. *J Med Educ.* 1974; **49**: 253–63.

10 Michaelson LK, Parmelee DX, McMahon KK, *et al. Team-Based Learning for Health Professions Education.* Sterling, VA: Stylus; 2008.

CHAPTER 9

Case studies in curriculum integration

This chapter outlines, in chronological sequence, four case studies, from the author's own experience, involving integration of a part or the whole of the undergraduate medical curriculum. In each case the author played a significant role in a change from a conventional discipline-based curriculum, or a part of it, to a more integrated one. The identity of the medical school involved in the change is withheld for reasons of confidentiality. Two of the attempts to change could be considered to have been successful, while the other two were not. The reasons for the success or failure of the change are analysed in relation to the guidelines for implementation of a change to an integrated curriculum described in Chapter 8.

CASE STUDY 1: SCHOOL A

The first study outlines an attempt to change a part of the preclinical curriculum to an integrated one from a strictly disciplinary one, on an experimental basis. The purpose of the experiment was to 'test the waters', in order to assess the desirability and feasibility of introducing integration across the whole of the preclinical curriculum. The experiment had a further purpose of exposing teachers to the concept and practicalities of integrated teaching, and students to those of integrated learning.

The medical school in which this experiment was carried out was a relatively young school that had inherited its curriculum from its much older parent school. The latter had a curriculum that had remained strictly discipline-based for decades, and was held in high esteem for the quality of its products both inside and outside the country. When the new school was inaugurated it was considered a branch of the parent school, and, for a while, teachers appointed to it were transferred from the latter. In fact the departments in the new school were considered sub-departments of the parent school in the initial stages. This arrangement changed after the first five years, with the new school gaining total independence from the older one. Subsequently, each of the two schools was incorporated into a separate university.

When independence of the new school was attained, a senior professor from the parent school was appointed as the new dean. Until then the dean of the latter school had remained as administrative Head of the new one. The new dean, though senior in years, had foresight about potential developments in medical education. One of his accomplishments was to create a unit of medical education that would keep abreast of developments in the field and advise the faculty on matters pertaining to the curriculum. The experiment on integration was carried out as a project of the newly established medical education unit.

The course coordinator first interviewed the Heads of the three preclinical departments to obtain their permission and support to carry out the study, as it involved their departments. Two of the Heads were agreeable and willing to support it, while the third stated he was against the concept of integration but would lend the support of his department. He was of the view that integration should really occur in the minds of the learners, and that exposing them to an integrated curriculum was 'spoon-feeding them an already digested diet'. A course for the experiment was agreed upon by the Heads and the dean's approval sought. The dean expressed his support for the experiment and gave his unqualified approval.

At the first meeting of volunteers for the experiment, they were oriented to the Kemp model of instructional unit design.[1] Topic areas were identified within the course, and volunteers were requested to select topic areas for developing general and specific learning objectives. These objectives, though submitted by individuals from each discipline, had to be justified at interdisciplinary meetings in terms of the requirements of a basic doctor. Such planning resulted in heightened awareness, among participating teachers, of the contributions that had hitherto been made by these departments. These were discussed at several subsequent meetings of the entire planning group, improved upon and accepted. After agreeing on the sequence in which the topics areas would be taught, and on the types of teaching activities in the course (small group discussion, tutorials, demonstrations and practical classes were identified as the main teaching methods, with lectures being kept to a minimum), the three department Heads worked out a timetable, limiting total time allocation to what had been allotted to the same content in previous years when taught on a disciplinary basis. At a later meeting of the group, members were oriented to some principles of adult learning, in particular those related to active learning, coordination between theory and practice and relevance. The course coordinator then worked out the unit schedule, the grouping of students and the allocation of preceptors.

The experiment was implemented when the next batch of students was admitted to the preclinical phase. Volunteer teachers, irrespective of their primary discipline, participated in the small group discussions, which integrated the relevant content while the practical classes and demonstrations were confined to disciplinary specialists.

Difficulties were experienced during the initial period, in particular the following four points.

1 Some teachers found it difficult to facilitate small group discussions that inevitably involved disciplines other than their own.

2 Some teachers tended to revert to didactism due to their uneasiness with facilitating small groups.

3 Inadequacy of time to 'cover' the identified objectives was a common concern.

4 Departments had difficulty in obtaining individual assessment scores for disciplines from an end-of-unit examination that combined all three disciplines.

The experiment was evaluated by seeking the perceptions of the key participants in it, using a questionnaire to students and interviews with teachers who participated. The latter was carried out immediately after the unit was implemented, while the questionnaire was administered to students more than a year later, after they had completed the preclinical examination. This delay was deliberate as it was felt that students would be more frank in expressing their opinions without the threat of an impending examination. Many aspects of the unit were evaluated, but only those results pertaining to the integrative nature of the unit will be dealt with here.

The majority of students favoured an integrated approach and agreed that joint participation by the three departments facilitated their learning. Students valued the synchronisation of teaching in this area among the three departments, as it facilitated learning of relationships. Teachers who participated in the experiment also vouched for its desirability and were of the view that it should be continued.

Monitoring of the experimental course was undertaken on a fortnightly basis and minor changes made depending on the feedback. A second group of students was exposed to the same course a year later, before summative evaluation of the first course could be undertaken. After the summative evaluation was completed its results were discussed at a meeting of the entire faculty. A significant change had occurred in the school's administration by now, as a new dean had been appointed to replace the previous one who was in favour of the experiment. The new dean was non-committal about the concept of integration and the value of the experiment. When the matter was discussed in the meeting, in spite of the fact that positive comments were made by most participants in the course, some trepidation in extending the concept to other areas of the preclinical curriculum was evident. At this point one of the three Heads of the preclinical departments (not the Head who was against integration in principle) made the astounding statement that his department was able to undertake teaching the entire course without the help of the other two departments. The new dean took this opportunity to rule that the future teaching of this course would be undertaken by the department whose Head was willing to do so alone. The whole idea of integration was thereby negated and the preclinical curriculum thereafter continued to be strictly discipline-oriented.

Lessons

➤ Introducing integration through an experiment may succeed in changing a curriculum if the experimental area forms a significant part of the curriculum. Procrastination in spreading the experiment to other areas in the second year may have been responsible for its ultimate failure.

➤ A delay in summative evaluation was the reason for this procrastination. Experimental courses such as this should be evaluated immediately and appropriate action taken to expand or curtail the experiment.

➤ The administrator, in this instance the dean, had an important role to play in the innovation. As the second dean was not committed to the innovation, steps should have been taken to win him over before the results of the experiment were discussed at a formal level.

➤ Some participants in the innovation may have had ulterior motives in accepting it. It was obvious that the Head of the department who volunteered to conduct the course solely in his department had either not understood the concept of integration or used the opportunity to obtain more curricular time and resources for his department.

CASE STUDY 2: SCHOOL B

This study is of an attempt to introduce curriculum integration in one of the oldest and most prestigious medical schools in a country that has had a long history of being influenced by developments in medical education. Under the guidance of a national body charged with the task, among others, of improving medical education in the country, a core curriculum for basic medical education was set up in collaboration with the deans of the several medical schools, with integration and community orientation as the cornerstones. However, there was considerable variation in both the manner and the degree to which the core curriculum was implemented in the various medical schools.

In the school under study the curriculum that existed before the development of the core curriculum was a conventional one, having been established several decades before the change to be described was instituted. A preclinical phase of three years consisted of normal basic sciences followed by 'abnormal' basic sciences, without any clinical exposure of the student to clinical studies. The clinical phase that followed, of three years' duration, included the major clinical specialities and sub-specialities, through clerkship rotations interspersed with didactic theoretical teaching. Consultative assistance was requested from experts in medical education to help the faculty plan an integrated curriculum, in line with the philosophy of the core curriculum. However, at a preliminary meeting of senior representatives of each department of the school and of the medical education unit, a reluctance to undertake a complete overhaul of the curriculum was apparent. Instead they agreed to undertake a pilot project in integration to determine its feasibility and, it was hoped, encourage its acceptance on a wider scale later on. Unlike in Case Study 1, however, agreement was reached to integrate the teaching that was currently taking place in one organ system across all the years of the curriculum, in a manner that would not interfere with the existing curricular or departmental structures.

An organ system was selected for the pilot project. Current teaching in this system was reviewed and a plan developed for integrating the teaching in each year at a horizontal level, but incorporating some amount of vertical integration to highlight relevance and applicability. The medical education unit, in collaboration with an interdisciplinary group, was given the responsibility of planning and coordinating the implementation of this project. The latter group consisted of nominated representatives from each of the departments, basic science and clinical, that contributed to teaching the selected system in the existing curriculum. The plan was accepted by faculty and implementation commenced shortly thereafter.

Further development of the practice of integration in the remaining parts of the curriculum did not occur over the next 10 years. At this time the school decided to introduce a problem-based curriculum. Unfortunately, the experience of implementing the latter was not a positive one, even though students who were exposed to it were equivocal about it. The innovation was abandoned after one year and though some degree of integration remained in the curriculum it had not occurred to a significant extent. Subsequent attempts were made to increase the degree of integration and, seven years after the attempt at problem-based learning, several integrated modules, particularly at a horizontal level, existed within the curriculum. The modules that displayed such integration were mostly in areas that did not impinge much on the content-oriented parts of the curriculum, indicative of reluctance on the part of strongly established departments to lose control of teaching and assessment. It is significant to note, in this respect, that in this country department Heads have an inordinate degree of autonomy and the dean's role is mostly administrative. Interdisciplinary committees tend to be overruled by departments on curricular matters and authorities have shown a reluctance to empower these committees to accept total responsibility for the integrated parts of the curriculum. Such departmental autonomy has also led to a reluctance of teachers to work together across departments. A lack of communication between basic science and clinical faculty was evident. There existed a distinct separation between these two groups as far as the curriculum was concerned, with the latter not considering the first two years of the curriculum as part of their domain and the former treating the last two years likewise. The situation was exacerbated by the inordinate workload of teachers, who were busily engaged in private practice in addition to their institutional responsibilities by way of service, teaching and administration.

Another factor that militated against an integrated curriculum in this country was the imposition, by the higher education authorities, of a credit point system that stipulated each type of teaching activity in relation to a given discipline. This requirement stifled curricular flexibility and hampered attempts at integration. Closely associated with this requirement was the system of student assessment, which was neither integrated nor problem-solving, and tested mainly the lower levels of cognition. Teachers were concerned that, if examinations became truly integrated, separate scores could not be assigned to the different disciplines, and this would adversely affect the nature of the transcripts that would be issued to graduates. This case was a good example of how bureaucratic procedures were given precedence over learning principles, whereas the former should be more concerned with the improvement of the curriculum.

Lessons

➤ As interdisciplinary committees were not given total responsibility for managing appropriate parts of the curriculum, and departmental Heads had control over their respective content areas for decision-making, the integrated curriculum was unlikely to have succeeded.

➤ The attempt at integration in the form of a pilot project, even if it spread across the curriculum, was likely to have been submerged by the major part of the curriculum that was discipline-based, unless there was a genuine need felt by the majority of the faculty for instituting an integrated curriculum.

➤ Bureaucratic procedures took precedence over learning strategies based on sound educational and curriculum principles, while the former should have been adapted to practices exemplifying the latter.

➤ Student assessment practices should have promoted integrated learning if the real effects of the integrated curriculum were to have been achieved.

CASE STUDY 3: SCHOOL C

This study is of a development that took place across the entire undergraduate medical curriculum in one of the oldest medical schools in the region. The school had for a long time followed a conventional curriculum that it had inherited from the colonial masters of the country in which it was situated. This curriculum earlier consisted of four phases – premedical, preclinical, paraclinical and clinical. The premedical phase, of one year's duration, consisted of disciplines considered prerequisite to the study of medicine (such as chemistry, physics and biology); the preclinical phase, of one and a half years' duration, consisted of the 'normal' basic sciences (anatomy, physiology and biochemistry); the paraclinical phase, of two years' duration, consisted of the 'abnormal' basic sciences (pathology, microbiology, parasitology, forensic medicine, pharmacology) as well as public health and junior clinical clerkships; the final clinical phase, of two years' duration, consisted of senior clerkship rotations in the major specialities and sub-specialities with didactic teaching in these same branches. Interdisciplinary integration, either at horizontal or vertical level, was minimal and incidental rather than deliberate. When the particular development described commenced the premedical year had long since been abandoned.

The school did not at first have a medical education unit of its own, although its teachers occasionally participated in the educational activities of a unit in a neighbouring medical school. Thereby some of them were exposed to global developments in medical education. It is apparent that, at one point in time, there was a growing body of teachers who were dissatisfied with the existing system of medical education in the school and were desirous of exploring the possibility of curriculum development. One senior department Head mooted the possibility of developing an integrated curriculum in the school and to this end inquired from a faculty member in an overseas medical education centre whether a group of senior professors could spend a period of time there developing plans for an integrated curriculum. When this visit eventuated, the faculty member undertook to spend two weeks full-time with this group, focusing on the specific objectives of the visit and facilitating activities leading to the accomplishment of its objectives.

The group was initially apprised of a competency-based model for developing an integrated unit of the curriculum. Thereafter, an organ system on which the group could practise developing an integrated module was selected. After the general objectives were agreed upon, the existing curriculum was reviewed by the group to determine which disease conditions related to the selected organ system were being dealt with in the existing curriculum. Discussion took place among the group as to omissions and irrelevancies in the current curriculum, bearing in mind the primary aim of the school, which was to produce a basic doctor for the needs of the country in which the school was situated. When agreement was reached, often after much animated discussion, the agreed list of conditions was categorised in a logical manner and allotted to each of several smaller interdisciplinary subgroups. These subgroups were required to follow the competency-based approach in deriving the content and specific objectives for the allotted areas, by working on their own under the guidance of the facilitator. When this work was completed after about five days of intensive activity, the products of each subgroup were presented to the entire group and discussed. After agreement was arrived at, methods for student achievement of the objectives in an integrated manner were discussed in general, by which time the two weeks had been exhausted. However, the group was now trained in undertaking a competency-based approach to curriculum development, which they were required to demonstrate to their colleagues in their home institution.

On return to the school interdisciplinary groups were set up for each of the organ systems and the method of deriving content demonstrated with the help of examples from the system that had been completed. The group, assisted by a medical education unit that had by now been set up, examined the curriculum as a whole and identified four streams within it: basic sciences, clinical sciences, behavioural sciences and community medicine. In the meantime each group continued to work on the system assigned to it. This activity, undoubtedly, took an inordinately long time, as this work was being undertaken in addition to the teaching, service and administrative commitments of the faculty members. Nevertheless, slowly but surely the work was completed. While working on these tasks the faculty decided, in keeping with developing trends in medical education, to introduce focal problems in each system. In addition, other forms of integrative methods were included in the curriculum plan. Realising the importance of student assessment, faculty now thought it was time to develop skills in student assessment procedures that would conform to the integrated curriculum.

A second group of teachers visited the same medical education centre as the first group and worked with the same facilitator to identify and develop skills in an appropriate system of student assessment for an integrated curriculum. A strategy for student assessment across the whole curriculum was agreed upon and presented to the rest of the faculty on the group's return home. This strategy was discussed and modified before it was accepted by faculty. At this stage the school organised a meeting, in a resort away from the school, for the entire faculty and consultants who were intimately associated with the project. At this meeting the curriculum was presented to the faculty and discussed openly.

It must be stated that curriculum planning and acceptance was not as smooth as this description makes them appear to be. There were strong objections from some quarters, in particular one basic science department, which insisted that its existing teaching programme should not be pruned. Compromises had to be made to prevent jeopardising the development, and to some extent this department had its way. This resistance had not abated even after several years since implementation.

The medical education unit and a few dedicated faculty members were largely responsible for the successful introduction of the new curriculum, which was a complete overhaul of the established one. Above all, however, without the unstinting support of a succession of deans this major undertaking would not have reached fruition.

The third stage of the development was determining a system of programme evaluation. This was undertaken with consultative help on site, even though the evaluation was planned and put in place after the new curriculum was implemented.

Lessons

The success of this case can be attributed to several factors, in keeping with some of the guidelines mentioned in Chapter 8.

➤ The dean at the time of the initiative, and his successors, were strongly supportive of the change.

➤ A committed interdisciplinary group of senior teachers was willing to be trained and continued to be committed to the change.

➤ On their return home they were able to involve a large sector of the faculty in the development, thereby creating a sense of ownership among the majority of the faculty.

➤ The willingness to compromise when faced with resistance, in spite of some decisions going against the grain of integration, prevented alienation of important sections of the school.

➤ A new but strong medical education unit was willing to spearhead the development and provide able leadership.

➤ Opportunities were provided for the entire faculty to discuss the change in many forums.

➤ Consultative assistance was sought, but the faculty ensured that such assistance was according to the needs identified by faculty, and not initiated by the consultants.

CASE STUDY 4: SCHOOL D

The final case study is the most recent, and involves a relatively young medical school in which a conventional curriculum had been operating for a few years. The majority of the teachers in this school were expatriate staff who had been trained themselves, and taught previously, in conventional, discipline-based curricula. The change was mooted by the dean and a senior member of faculty who had gained some exposure to the field of medical education.

A medical education unit was set up in the school, under the dean as chair and supported by three faculty members, with a remit to support faculty in their roles as teachers. The school hosted an international conference in medical education, to which were invited educators from other medical schools in the region. All faculty members were requested to review the existing curriculum, identify any deficient areas and suggest methods to correct these deficiencies. The feasibility of synchronising related components of the existing curriculum was studied by the unit, but it was concluded that integration of the curriculum would result in a patchwork without any sense of direction.

A workshop was now organised, to develop a new integrated model, led by a medical educationist from another school. From this workshop a conceptual model for a revised curriculum emerged. A curriculum task force mapped out the contents and related activities for the premedical phase of the curriculum, which consisted of four modules. This was discussed by the entire faculty and, though no consensus was reached, the majority agreed on the need for an integrated curriculum. A consultant was invited to develop a sample model and, at a workshop, the phases and broad content areas of the new curriculum were agreed upon. A sample module developed by workshop participants under the consultant's guidance served as a template for developing other modules.

Organ-system module committees attempted to develop the contents of the first two phases of the curriculum based on the sample module, but did not find the activity productive, and issues raised by faculty were resolved at a plenary discussion led by the consultant. A second workshop convened to develop modules was more productive, and the consultant worked closely with individual committees to complete outlines for each module. The organ-system module committees were reconstituted to be more representative of content areas identified in each module, and these committees were given the responsibility of identifying teaching strategies and resources for their respective modules. Throughout this process the medical education unit facilitated the activities of the module committees.

Faculty development workshops on specific topics, such as problem-based learning, were conducted *pari passu* with curriculum development. All faculty members were involved in these activities. The modules developed were reviewed by the consultant with the respective module coordinators, and suggestions made for improvement. A coordinator for the first phase of the curriculum was appointed to oversee and coordinate the work of the module committees in that phase.

At the next stage a workshop on integrated teaching and assessment was conducted by the consultant for all faculty members. At this workshop participants identified appropriate teaching strategies for the first phase of the curriculum, and developed skills in constructing assessment items that would enhance integrated learning in keeping with the philosophy of the new curriculum. In addition, progress made in planning the new curriculum was reviewed.

At this stage a committee to review the third (clinical) phase of the curriculum was formed, to identify inadequacies of the existing clinical teaching programme and suggest remedial measures and teaching strategies in keeping with the new integrated curriculum. The medical education unit conducted a meeting of all clinical faculty members to inform them of the progress made with the new curriculum as a prelude to planning the clinical phase. In the meantime a six-day workshop for all faculty members was held to draft the new curriculum for the first two phases. This draft included, for each module, the aims, intended learning outcomes, key skills, methods of teaching and learning including physical and time resources and an outline of a typical week. This work took longer than had been anticipated and faculty members worked for a further 10 days to complete the curriculum document. This document was reviewed by the consultant who, in conjunction with each module coordinator, made necessary adjustments to the draft document.

It was time now to address in greater depth the clinical phase of the curriculum. Clinical committees for each speciality and sub-speciality were constituted, and the chair of the medical education unit oriented clinical faculty to the curricular reforms that were by now being implemented in the school. This orientation was considered necessary because of the high turnover of clinical teachers in the school. Following a presentation to clinical teachers by the same consultant, clinical committees worked on their respective areas and the ensuing curricular documents were submitted for perusal by the medical education unit.

The consultant advised the school authorities that the success of the new curriculum would ultimately depend on the manner in which it was implemented, rather than the quality of the curriculum plan that was documented. Successful implementation would depend on the degree to which faculty members were trained to implement the integrative practices that the plan envisaged. While some faculty development had already taken place through short workshops, it was necessary to develop a group of faculty members who had a deeper understanding of, and more skills in, sound educational practices. An extended programme of faculty development was suggested and accepted by the school authorities. In order to reward busy faculty members who were willing to pursue such training, a diploma was to be awarded to those who successfully completed the programme. This programme was planned and implemented in conjunction with the introduction of the new curriculum. Whenever possible, the emphasis within this programme was the new medical curriculum, and participants were oriented towards planning, implementing and evaluating integrated curricula and courses.

Implementation of the new curriculum commenced almost six years after the feasibility of integrating the first two phases of the curriculum was first discussed, and five years after serious planning of an integrated curriculum started. A core group for programme evaluation had been formed before implementation commenced and had undertaken planning for evaluation by the time the first batch of students was exposed to the new programme. As part of the faculty development programme, methods for evaluation of the new curriculum were emphasised, and some participants selected this topic as their research project.

The first students who were subjected to the programme were closely monitored. To the great satisfaction of the faculty, these students' perceptions of the new curriculum were very positive, encouraging faculty to further develop the concept of integration. An accreditation team visiting the school also evaluated the new curriculum positively. The integrated curriculum continues to be implemented in this school.

Lessons

➤ The initiation of the project by the dean and the support given to it by his successors were crucial to the success of the new curriculum.

➤ The commitment and ownership of the new curriculum, created by the involvement of all faculty members in one way or another, facilitated the development.

➤ In spite of a fairly high turnover of teachers in this school, the creation of a critical mass of trained and committed individuals among them ensured that the curriculum would not in any way be diverted from its original philosophy.

➤ The prior creation of a medical education unit enabled overall responsibility for the curriculum to be vested in its members, who were willing, in spite of their busy schedules, to provide continuity to the project.

➤ The strategy of training faculty, both by workshops and in a diploma programme, in course planning, teaching methods, student assessment methods and programme evaluation methods, *pari passu* with the planning and implementation of the new curriculum, facilitated the 'curriculum in action' to conform to the 'curriculum on paper'.

➤ Regular visits by the same consultant at reasonably spaced yet well-timed intervals provided continuity and encouragement to the faculty in seeing the project through.

➤ Positive comments by both students and external evaluators greatly encouraged faculty in maintaining the innovation.

ANALYSIS OF THE FOUR CASE STUDIES

In this section the four case studies are compared. They are arranged, in the author's opinion, in a sequence that demonstrates increasing degrees of successful outcomes. While this fact may be a reflection of increasing experience in curriculum development, it enables one to surmise as to what it is that makes an innovation, such as curriculum integration, work. The four strategies will be compared to identify tendencies from the studies taken as a group.

As case studies by their very nature are situation-specific, it is difficult to extrapolate findings from one study to another situation. This difficulty may be partly overcome through a series of case studies from which generalisations may be drawn. The number of case studies in the series described is, however, too small for deriving generalisations, and one can only point out tendencies, which would have to be verified further through an accumulation of similar studies.

The first two cases (Schools A and B) demonstrated the futility of attempting to introduce an innovation through an experimental approach if the initial experiment is not extended immediately thereafter to a larger part of the curriculum. In the first, the experiment was limited to a single unit of study within a large phase of the curriculum, while in the second it was limited to a single organ system throughout the entire curriculum. In both instances, the experiment was not extended to other parts of the curriculum.

The author is a proponent of the experimental strategy for introducing educational innovations and is wary of complete curriculum overhaul. He has witnessed several schools reject an innovation because of the insistence on the latter strategy in the face of considerable faculty resistance. Howard Barrows, an eminent medical educationist and a strong proponent of the practice of problem-based learning in medical education, once indicated to the author that he was against the experimental strategy because the segment of the curriculum included in the experiment was often 'submerged' by the remainder of the curriculum (personal communication, 1987). The experience of the first two cases tends to lend credence to this argument.

A significant problem in the first two cases, and one that perhaps led to their failure to spread the innovation to the rest of the curriculum, was the fact that a critical mass of protagonists of the innovation had not been created in the respective schools at the time the experiment started, or during its implementation. In School A this problem was confounded by the delay in obtaining student feedback about the experience and, in the meantime, the appointment of a new dean who was not committed to the concept of integration. In School B the few protagonists were diluted by a large segment of faculty who were either against or equivocal about integration. In both schools the innovators were hopeful that the skills and positive attitudes gained by some teachers would maintain and even extend the innovation, but they underestimated the power of antagonists in thwarting its spread.

In Schools C and D a strategy of complete curriculum overhaul was successful in implementing and maintaining the innovation. In both schools, however, the involvement of at least the majority, if not all, of the teachers in planning the innovation was a critical factor in its success. While in School C there was a small segment of the faculty who voiced their opposition to integration, the willingness to compromise facilitated successful implementation. In both, strong and active support by the administration ensured its introduction and maintenance.

These case studies have demonstrated how difficult it is, and how long it takes, to bring about significant curricular innovation. Yet the positive outcomes of the attempts in the latter two schools should encourage innovators and provide guidance as to how to maximise the chances of introducing and maintaining an integrated curriculum successfully.

KEY POINTS

- If an experimental strategy is used to introduce curriculum integration, the experiment should be evaluated immediately and steps taken to extend it, before the experiment is 'submerged' by the rest of the curriculum.
- Involvement of as many as possible of the implementers in planning the innovation is likely to enhance ownership and commitment to the plan.

- When a complete overhaul of the curriculum is attempted, innovators must be willing to compromise when significant and justifiable objections are raised.
- Significant curriculum change is difficult and time-consuming, but positive outcomes are encouraging.

REFERENCE

1 Kemp JE. *Instructional Design: a plan for unit and course development.* Belmont, CA: Fearon; 1971.

Index

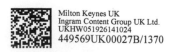

9 781846 195105